Two Thumbs Up

for your future in Orofacial myology.

Chris Mills

Two Thumbs Up

*Awareness, Education, and Treatment
of Thumb Sucking*

*A Guide for
Parents and Professionals*

Christine Stevens Mills B.S., SLP, COM™
IAOM Certified Orofacial Myologist™
Speech/Language Pathologist

Copyright © 2006
All rights reserved.

Registration Number: TXu001283045
Date: 2006-02-21

ISBN - 9781548924256

DEDICATION

This book is dedicated to a special lady who was not only a consummate professional, a colleague, a mentor, and the person who encouraged me to move forward with writing this book, she was my life-long friend Anita Weinfield.

I recall we were both at an IAOM convention in Philadelphia. At the end of a long conference day, we decided to unwind in the lobby bar and order martinis. While sipping on our drinks, I brought up my idea of writing this book and wanted her opinion. I can still hear her voice. She did more than encourage me to write it. She said, "I had to write it, or else!" And if you knew Anita, you knew she was not a force to be reckoned with. Her recent passing left great sadness, however, her words of encouragement and warm friendship will always embrace me. Thank You Anita!

Acknowledgment

'RYAN AND HIS FRIEND' ~ ARTWORK ~ COURTESY OF NANCY RUPPERT

PROOFREADING AND EDITING ~ A SPECIAL THANK YOU TO CONNIE BROTZKE

A VERY SPECIAL THANK YOU

FORMATTING, PROOFREADING, EDITING, PHOTOGRAPHS AND SUPPORT
MY HUSBAND ~ GALEN R. MILLS

CONTENTS

1	The Pathway to Success	1
2	What Every Parent Should Know	5
3	Story: Ryan and his Friend	17
4	Prepare for a Thumb Program	25
5	Sample Step by Step Thumb Program	41
6	The Professional Connection	57
7	Positive Effects of Thumb Sucking	75
8	Laughter Makes us Healthier	81
9	Case Studies	85
10	Resources	101

Throughout this book I will utilize selective words for efficient clarification. When referencing male, female, adolescent, adult, patient or the gender pronouns he or she, all will be referred to as 'child'. Although the information is relevant to mothers, fathers, grandparents and caregivers, I will refer to all as 'mother'. Despite using the title, '*Two Thumbs Up*, thumb, finger and tongue sucking can be equally detrimental and necessary to address, therefore, finger and tongue sucking will be referred to as 'thumb sucking'.

Chapter 1

The Pathway to Success

Thumb Sucking is not a simple habit, but a multi-faceted complex pattern that can affect mind and body. Thumb sucking is generally perceived as a 'simple habit', something not to be concerned with, having little or no ramifications, or when ready, the thumb sucker will simply stop... or will he?

Neuroscience explains pleasurable activities stimulate the brain to produce chemicals called neurotransmitters communicating information throughout the brain and body. The action of thumb sucking releases inhibitory neurotransmitters producing the feelings of pleasure and comfort. This action/reaction reinforces the behavior, neural pathways form connecting perception/reaction and repetition deepens the pathway with similar stimulus becoming a learned behavior.

Multiple body complications may also develop such as: changes in the oro-facial structure and developing malocclusions, changes in breathing patterns from nasal breathing to oral respiration, changes in rest posture of the tongue and lips, changes in speech. I could go on and on.

I have been in private practice for over forty years treating thumb sucking patterns. The questions that parents ask most frequently are:

- "Why wasn't I told earlier that thumb sucking could and would do damage to my child's teeth?"

- "Why wasn't I told there was someone like you to help my child stop sucking his thumb?"

- "Why isn't there educational information about thumb sucking complications in the dentist's, orthodontist's, or pediatrician's office?"

Throughout my career, these questions have constantly been raised by parents when they arrive with their child for a consultation. A pivotal moment occurred, when a pediatrician brought his child for treatment of a severe thumb sucking problem. It was surprising that a professional, who works with children and their health issues, knew nothing about the consequences of thumb sucking. It was then that I knew I had to write this book for the thumb sucking child, parent and professional. There are many thumb sucking books available, but I wanted mine to specifically address the following:

Desire + Awareness + Education = Successful Treatment

Desire - I want the parent and thumb sucker to understand the desire to stop thumb sucking needs to come from the thumb sucker himself. I want the thumb sucker to understand there is help available. Desire to stop and the willingness to try is the first step.

Awareness - I want the child, parent and professional to be aware there is help for the thumb sucker. There are many available choices of treatment. One treatment plan does not fit all. A positive therapeutic plan that successfully eliminates their habit without anxiety, fear or pain is available. Thumb sucking elimination should and can be a fun, positive experience for all involved. There are professionals with specialized training to help eliminate thumb sucking. The International Association of Orofacial Myology, being one of these, will have a list of qualified therapists and information on how to locate one in your area at www.iaom.com.

Education - I would like the reader to be aware that thumb sucking is, 'more than just a simple habit.' Recognizing thumb sucking can result in physical changes, as well as, have emotional and or social ramifications is a critical first step. Knowledge and understanding will allow the reader to apply this new awareness allowing the recipient to interpret and process possibilities, expand insight which expand decision-making. Information cannot be converted into knowledge without education.

Health care specialists and allied health care professionals are key to total patient care. I have dedicated a section to 'The Professional Connection' (Chapter 6) highlighting the complexity of thumb sucking and the diverse complications that affect their clientele. By clarifying the actions and consequences of thumb sucking along with pointing out the benefits of thumb sucking elimination parent and child will understand this step is necessary to create a stable environment for the treatment protocol with the ultimate goal of health and well-being for the child.

This section also provides tools that can be utilized prior to and or during child and parent consultation. This didactic, informative section will be an asset to the office library. This book will help focus attention on potential thumb sucking problems, the child and parents may not be aware of, encouraging dialogue on the subject.

Also included in this section for therapeutic professionals who may wish to address thumb sucking is a step by step treatment protocol, helpful hints, pitfalls to avoid and many other ideas I have developed and/or refined over the past forty years.

Children, parents and professionals are all equally important to a successful thumb elimination program. The format of the book was designed to visualize, connect, and empower the reader.

I have always believed knowledge empowers us to see with clarity. A personal phrase I have used throughout my career says it all, "If you do not know it, you will not see it. If you cannot see it, you cannot treat it." Which brings us to my winning formula for successful thumb sucking elimination: **Desire** leads to **Awareness** which leads to **Education** resulting in successful **Treatment**. This has been my winning formula for successful thumb sucking elimination for forty years in private practice. I now would like to share this winning formula with you.

Making the Connection
The pathway to success comes from within. Most individuals want to feel in control, self-confident and successful. Thumb sucking diminishes all three of these feelings. Success with any endeavor is best achieved with a plan. *Two Thumbs Up* helps provide that plan.

Chapter 2

What Every Parent Should Know

First, the thumb sucker and parent need to have the **DESIRE** to become **AWARE** of the consequences of thumb sucking. Then the child needs to be **EDUCATED** on how to help themselves eliminate this pattern. And lastly, the child needs to be motivated to achieve successful **TREATMENT.**

When Does Thumb Sucking Start?

For some children thumb sucking starts pre-birth. We have all seen an ultrasound image of a baby sucking their thumb while still in the womb. These first images are precious. And, thumb sucking continues to be viewed as an endearing behavior even after baby arrives. Some babies put their thumb in their mouth, some suck on their fingers, some even put their whole fist in their mouth as they learn to utilize the sucking action necessary for survival. So, at this early stage, thumb sucking is considered natural and necessary and at this point, there is very little need for concern. When this sucking action occurs between feedings, it then can be considered a supplemental reward and gratification. Generally, the thumb sucking pattern will lessen or cease between the ages of three and four. Beyond that age, thumb sucking can cause real damage to the dentition (teeth) and other oro-facial structures. (The related specifics will be discussed later in this text.)

Moving to the other end of the spectrum...

When Does Thumb Sucking Stop?

The answer may be never...! Once baby is walking and talking, thumb sucking should diminish or stop altogether. When it does not, the child has most likely linked thumb sucking to a feeling of comfort, a safe feeling...such as being held in a blanket by a loving mother. Some children eventually wean themselves off thumb sucking much the same way they are weaned off the bottle. Others, however, continue the pattern for years. When they do so, we say that thumb sucking has become a 'set behavior'. And, once the behavior is set, it becomes difficult to stop.

Older children and adult thumb suckers learn to hide the behavior from others and suck only when they are alone, watching TV, reading, resting and sleeping. In my professional career, I have treated thumb suckers in their twenties and beyond. At this age, the individual is very hesitant to seek help.

While the behavior seems harmless enough, it is important to get to the cause of the behavior. Has it become a set pattern established through frequent use or, in fact, is it a deeply rooted psychological problem? Often, the older child, teen or adult thumb sucker may suffer low self-esteem or real embarrassment to still be sucking their thumb at their age. Additionally, there are many physiological harms which can result from thumb sucking and will be discussed later in this book.

Once thumb sucking has become a set pattern, it becomes crucial to determine what has triggered that pattern. In other words, it is important to learn if the behavior is an established pattern due to frequent use or if it is due to some deep-seated emotional underpinnings. If the pattern has become set due to an emotional problem, the help of a psychiatrist, psychologist or counselor may be in order. In general, however, thumb sucking is an established pattern, something that is habitual and may be corrected. But don't underestimate the power of this established pattern.

There are some physiological changes that may occur that make this pattern difficult to break. In a word, the attractiveness is due to **endorphins**. Most of us have heard of endorphins as they relate to exercise and health. By definition endorphins are any of a group of hormones secreted within the brain and nervous system causing an analgesic effect. We think of an endorphin rush as it relates to strenuous physical activity or as a reaction to the physical attractiveness of others. But, did you know that thumb sucking produces an increase in endorphins in the brain thus causing a feeling of comfort and pleasure? What is the harm of that, you are thinking. Hold on. We will get to that. But for starters, think about what might happen to your standing in the community if you walked around with your thumb in your mouth.

Consider what thumb sucking can do to the skin on your thumb and the shape of your mouth. The persistent sucking pattern can also have effects on your teeth.

Going back to the endorphin rush, in children and sometimes young adults, this feeling of comfort can be very powerful. The thumb sucking may calm the child down, giving the individual that comfortable safe feeling while also allowing the child to tune out, becoming more sedate. Many parents may feel they need not be concerned with the thumb sucking pattern because the thumb sucker is not having tantrums, hurting himself or being disruptive. However, the thumb sucking increases the endorphins leading to more thumb sucking. And, yes, more thumb sucking leads to more endorphins, which leads to still more thumb sucking. And so, the habitual merry-go-round continues.

Some children cannot seem to get to sleep without sucking their thumb. This sucking helps to relax them so that they can get to sleep. If the sucking action is slight and the thumb falls out of the mouth once asleep, it is likely that little harm will occur, and, in this particular case, intervention may not be necessary. However, if the sucking action is very strong there can be a great deal of damage, in this case, intervention is essential.

Thumb Sucking - What Age to Stop?
The opinion of the American Dental Association (ADA), as well as, the American Academy of Pediatrics (AAP) is that a child should generally stop thumb sucking by the age of three. Prior to that they feel little or no damage will occur from thumb sucking. Their general opinion is that only after the age of three significant problems with the teeth or jaw line may occur. However, parents **remember** this formula:

**Frequency + Intensity + Duration =
Amount of Damage**

If your child is constantly sucking their thumb, the sucking action is intense or if your child has been sucking since birth, you probably will see damage occurring to the teeth long before age three. If your child only places their thumb lightly in their mouth while falling asleep and it falls out of their mouth when they fall asleep, there may be little or no damage occurring.

The Pacifier - Thumbs Up or Down

When an individual is referred to me to treat a thumb sucking pattern, one of the most frequently asked questions by the parent during the initial consultation, is in regard to, pacifiers.
Is the pacifier better or worse than sucking the thumb? Should I have given the pacifier to my child instead of allowing the thumb sucking? Should I have taken the pacifier away at an earlier age? When these questions are presented to me I get a flash back to when I was pregnant with my son. As a prospective new mother, I had the same concerns and read a great deal about babies, talked to friends who already had children and still needed answers about thumb sucking and pacifiers.

One of the most interesting and eye-opening conversations came from one of my best friends who had two children. Because we had been friends for so long she was very knowledgeable of my profession and we had talked extensively about thumb sucking. One day over lunch she brought up the topic of pacifiers. She asked me what I thought of pacifiers and was one type of pacifier better for a child than another? I proceeded to give her my expert advice regarding what I had learned about the shape of pacifiers and which shape was supposed to be better for a child. In those days the NUK exerciser was the pacifier of choice compared to one with an elongated nipple which would extend further into the throat than the short squatty NUK. However, you need to know the shapes and textures of pacifiers and procedures in the hospital continue to change.

Continuing with my story, my friend looked at me and said, "Did you know that after the baby is born and is placed in the nursery the nurse immediately places a pacifier in the infant's mouth? That is standard protocol at most hospitals." I was shocked! I placed this information in my mind's vault for future reference. I had to open the vault earlier than I expected because a few weeks later my son arrived early. As the nurse was wheeling me down the corridor to have the baby I recall speaking in a matter-of-fact tone of voice, "Put it on my chart, NO PACIFIER!" As it turned out, I was happy with my decision. Even though he was three weeks early and only five pounds, he learned to suck just fine. He never needed a pacifier and never sucked his thumb.

Decide for Yourself

The formula Frequency + Intensity + Duration = Damage can also apply to the use of pacifiers. The decision whether to use a pacifier or not is up to you.

The Pros:
- A pacifier may soothe a fussy baby.
- A pacifier offers temporary distraction.
- A pacifier may help your baby go to sleep.
- Pacifiers are disposable.
- A pacifier may help reduce the risk of sudden infant death syndrome (SIDS) according to the American Academy of Pediatrics.

The Cons:
- Early pacifier use may interfere with breast feeding. Breast feeding is different from sucking on a pacifier. Some babies have trouble learning to breast feed if the pacifier is introduced too early. According to the AAP, if you plan on breast feeding, it is recommended you wait until the infant is one-month old before introducing the pacifier.
- The infant may become dependent on the pacifier.
- Continued use of the pacifier may lead to dental problems.

What is the Harm of Thumb Sucking?

Here are some additional considerations to help you determine if thumb sucking is a passing fancy or a set pattern. When I see how many young people are wearing braces today, I can't help but believe they might have benefited from thumb sucking intervention during their childhood. Let me explain:

The pressure of the thumb can contribute to many of the following problems related to the oro-facial structure
- The pressure of the thumb against the palate (roof of the mouth) can help to produce a high, narrow, arched palate which is not conducive to the proper rest posture for the tongue.
- The pressure and placement of the thumb in the mouth, along with the sucking action, can contribute to a misalignment of the dentition (teeth).
- The structure and appearance of the lips can change due to chronic thumb sucking.
- Thumb sucking forces the tongue to rest low and forward and during the sucking action the tongue moves forward in a thrusting action against the teeth. If this sucking continues, it encourages an inappropriate tongue posture for all oral functions and it is this related poor muscle function of all the muscles that is so detrimental to growth and development of the face.

Illustrating the damage that can occur from prolonged thumb sucking:

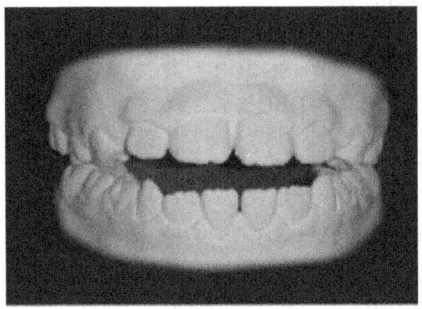

OPEN BITE

This **open-bite** (top and bottom teeth not coming together) often is created from prolonged thumb sucking. The photo illustrates how the thumb can act like a wedge holding the top and bottom teeth apart. Until you remove the thumb from the equation, the teeth are not allowed to grow and develop properly, therefore, creating a little window. This little window allows the tongue to rest in this space which also contributes to the malocclusion.

This **excessive overjet** (protruding top teeth-often called overbite) illustrates how the thumb sucking action places a great deal of pressure on the dentition forcing the top teeth to protrude. This position of the teeth makes it difficult to maintain natural lip closure.

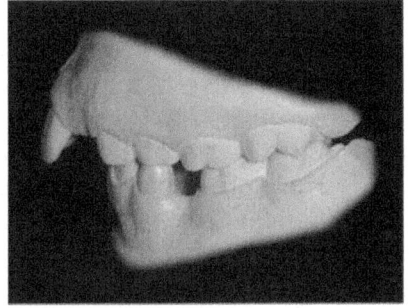

OVERJET

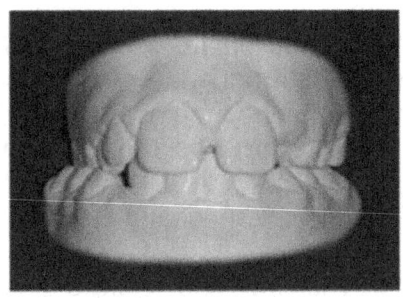

CROSS-BITE

Cross-bite: Strong thumb sucking action can contribute to another type of malocclusion called cross-bite. In simple terms the posterior teeth do not fit properly on one or both sides. The top teeth bite inside of the lower ones instead of outside as they should. This often causes the jaw to shift to one side when the person bites together.

The photo right illustrates a **normal shaped palate.** The horseshoe shape accommodates better spacing for the teeth and room for the tongue.

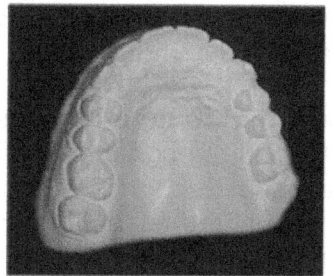

NORMAL PALATE

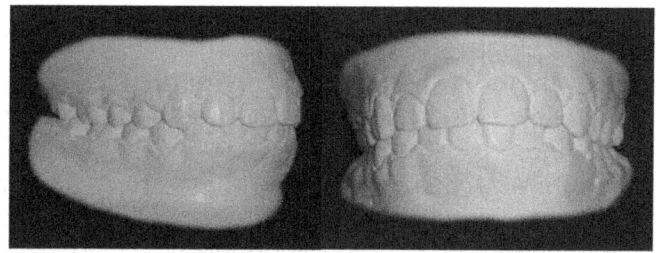

NORMAL OCCLUSION - The teeth meet harmoniously

Change in Tongue Posture
- When the tongue posture remains low and forward the jaw drops causing the lips to part.
- When the tongue rests low and forward and the lips remain parted the breathing patterns change from functional nasal breathing to an open mouth breathing pattern.
- This open mouth breathing pattern contributes to weakness of the orbicularis oris (muscles surrounding the lips). Lip strength is important because the lips are your natural retainer or maintainer of the teeth.
- The low forward rest posture of the tongue allows an incorrect spring off point for articulation, causing the sounds to be misarticulated.

Changes in Breathing Patterns
Ever body part is connected, and one body part will affect other parts of the body compensating by adapting when complications or trauma occur creating a snow ball effect of symptoms and problems

that need to be identified. Thumb sucking is one etiology that contributes to mouth breathing yet overlooked or not recognized.

Constant mouth breathing triggers the following effects
- Breathing through the mouth can contribute to gingivitis.
- Breathing through the mouth does not allow filtering of germs. Instead of the nose filtering germs and allergens, the individual is breathing in germs and allergens through the mouth and right into the lungs without a filter.
- Mouth breathing bypasses the nasal mucosa and can lead to nasal mucosa swelling which usually renders regular breathing difficult.
- Mouth breathing during sleep can contribute to loud snoring and irregular breathing. What you do during waking hours generally carries over into sleep. (Reference Mason).
- Interference with the preparation of inspired air for the lungs, increasing a child's vulnerability to upper respiratory infections.
- There is an increase in airflow volume when exhalation is accomplished through the mouth. When mouth breathing carbon-dioxide is expelled rapidly the body's normal oxygen absorption ability is diminished. When the exchange of oxygen and carbon dioxide is efficient, as with nasal breathing, the blood remains in a balanced chemical (pH) state. This balance serves to regulate and control cell activities that involve the body's metabolism.
- Mouth breathing effects the posture of the jaws, tongue, head, and occlusion, changing the normal posture. If mouth breathing becomes constant the growth consequences may include a longer face and dental changes.
- Breathing through your mouth can contribute to chronic chapped lips and licking of your lips.

Special Note:
Nasal breathing is critical to our health and overall well-being. 'The changes in breathing patterns' listed above highlight the many mouth breathing complications referred to as 'a snow ball effect'.

Being an advocate of 'Total Patient Care' I would be remiss if I didn't include this special note about Pediatric Sleep Apnea (PSA). When a child retains a constant mouth breathing pattern unidentified complications may be present. PSA, a type of Obstructive Sleep Disorders (OSA) being one of them.

Today, Pediatric Sleep Apnea (PSA) has become a major concern due to the potential life-long complications. Laymen associate OSA with adults and being overweight. We are learning our mouth breathing children also need to be evaluated for PSA. Pediatric sleep apnea complications can develop at an early age and cause complications throughout life.

Changes in Rest Posture of Lips and Tongue

A low and forward rest posture of the tongue, a bowed upper lip, and weak flaccid lower lip (below) illustrate the changes in rest posture of the tongue due to the thumb anchoring the tongue down during the thumb sucking action.

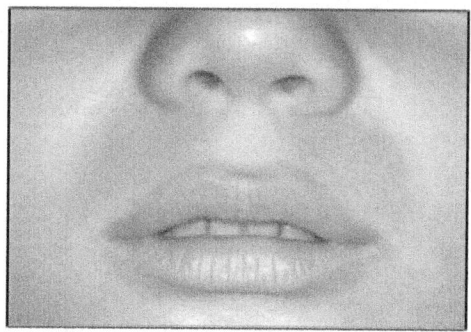

BOWED UPPER LIP

The bowed (rolling up) upper lip left illustrates changes in the lip structure due to the upper lip resting on the thumb. The weak flaccid lower lip illustrates weakness occurring due to the upper and lower lip not resting together naturally.

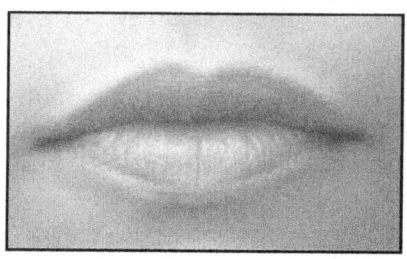

NORMAL LIPS

Is this Child Ready for the Program?

Most importantly, intervention should start only after you are sure that the individual child is in good physical, emotional, and psychological health, with no other problems that might distract from therapy.

Do Not Start a Program
- If there are health or psychological problems. Have the family deal with those first.
- If the family is in transition or in crisis (examples: illness, divorce, new baby, or moving).
- During the holidays.
- If both parents are not in agreement about intervention.

Not Ready to Stop Thumb Sucking

If, while attempting to stop, your child becomes a **flip-flopper** going back and forth...sucking, not sucking, sucking, not sucking, not consistently following directions, the child is not ready to stop. If the child is not willing to cooperate or work on the problem. The willingness to **TRY** is key; it helps to create confidence which is essential and imperative to SUCCESS.

When the child is first asked, "Do you want to stop sucking your thumb?" You may get a response like this...
"I don't want to stop."
"I don't know if I want to stop."
"I don't think I can stop."

This is a very normal first response. This child may be afraid they can't stop, so it is easier to say I don't want to stop. They also do not know what trying to stop entails. Remember the unknown is always scary. Explain we will work at this, as a team, we will have fun, the family will have to do silly stuff, and there is a reward system in place. This sounds less scary than the unknown - Right!

Ask and discuss these questions. Listen to your child's answers. The answers will provide insight to their thoughts and feelings. If you think they are ready, willing and able to cooperate, then it is time to make some decisions!

Ask these questions to see if the child is ready

yes/no	Would you like to try to stop sucking your thumb?
yes/no	Do you know why it is healthy for you to stop sucking your thumb?
yes/no	Do you think the thumb is doing damage to your teeth?
yes/no	Do you wash your hands before you suck your thumb?

yes/no	Do you hold a pillow, blanket, or stuffed animal when you suck your thumb?
yes/no	Are you being teased by others when you suck your thumb?
yes/no	Are you embarrassed to spend the night at a friend's home because you are afraid they will find out you suck your thumb?
yes/no	Do you want to grow up and have straight teeth or crooked teeth? (I usually hold up a mirror for the child to look at their teeth, and then I show them two pictures of teeth, one with a malocclusion and one with beautiful occlusion.) Then I ask which set of teeth would you like to have?
yes/no	While sucking, do you pull or twirl hair, chew on clothes, etc.?

ASK - Do You Want to Stop Sucking Your Thumb?
If the answer is: "**No**"

STOP!

Your child is **Not** ready to begin a Thumb Program. You need to wait a little while longer until your child says…

"**Yes**, I am READY to TRY!"

When the answer is **Yes**…

Praise your child for making this decision, then ask, "Why do you want to stop sucking your thumb?" Explain, "There is no right or wrong answer". "I want to understand this important decision from your perspective".

In my experience, when you listen to your child's answers you not only gain insight to their feelings and fears, you will know if your child is ready to stop thumb sucking.

Your Child Is Ready to Stop
- When your child agrees, "I am willing to try and stop."
- When your child can express why they want to stop.
- When your child states, "I am willing to follow the rules and directions."

Please read "**Ryan and his Friend**" with your child when you hear those words, *"Yes, I Am Ready to Try."*

Chapter 3

Ryan and his Friend

The story you are about to read will probably sound very familiar. Every thumb sucker at some point in time will have encountered one or more of the experiences portrayed in the story below. Most likely, with guided questions, the child will grasp an understanding of how Ryan feels by being transported into his world.

Through this journey Ryan comes to the realization that he wants to stop sucking his thumb and he asks for help. Reading this story with accompanying guided questions may navigate your child to the same decision. Asking questions are the simplest and most effective way of learning. Questions are the best way to gain insight. Insight into this particular undertaking encourages the Desire to begin his/her own journey.

Remember:

DESIRE + AWARENESS + EDUCATION = SUCCESS

A Thumb Sucker's Day

Ryan turns off his alarm clock and rolls onto his side. He puts his thumb back into his mouth and closes his eyes.

"Wake up, Sleepy Head. It's time to get out of bed," his mother calls cheerfully.

But Ryan feels warm and safe. The thumb in his mouth is a comfortable old friend. He ignores his mother's voice and soon is fast asleep.

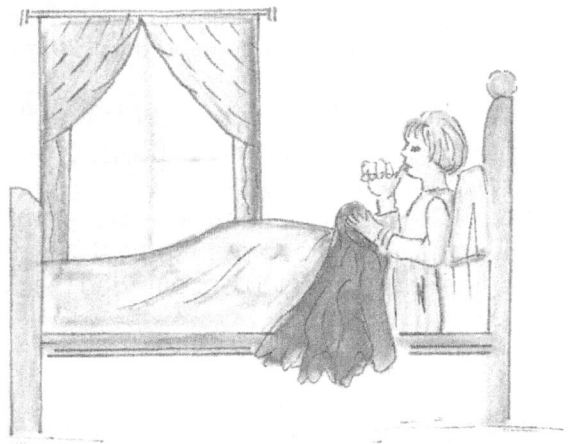

Clearly losing her temper with an edge of irritation in her voice, Ryan's mother shouts, "Ryan you need to get moving. You'll be late for school!" Reluctantly, Ryan gets up and gets dressed. He barely has time to eat his breakfast before running out to catch the bus.

Once seated on the school bus, Ryan's thumb finds its way back into his mouth. The other children notice Ryan sucking his thumb and they taunt him. They call him "thumb sucker" and "a baby". Some even mock him by sticking their thumbs into their mouths to show him how ridiculous he looks. One boy asks him if he has a 'blankie' in his backpack. Ryan pulls his thumb out of his mouth, but the teasing has only made him want to suck his thumb more. His thumb, after all, is a faithful friend who never teases. Long before he reaches school, the thumb is back in Ryan's mouth.

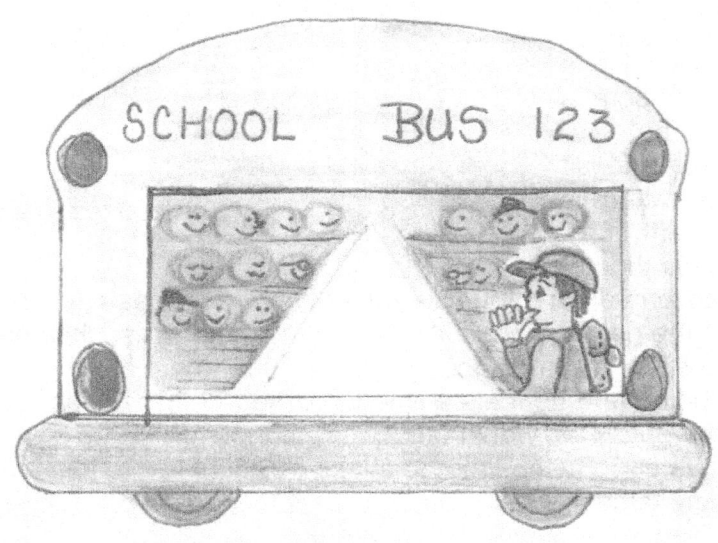

Ryan's class has been learning about marine life. Mrs. Brotzke, his favorite teacher, is pointing to a picture of a dolphin and she tells the class, "Today we are going to learn about dolphins and sharks. They are each an important part of our eco system."

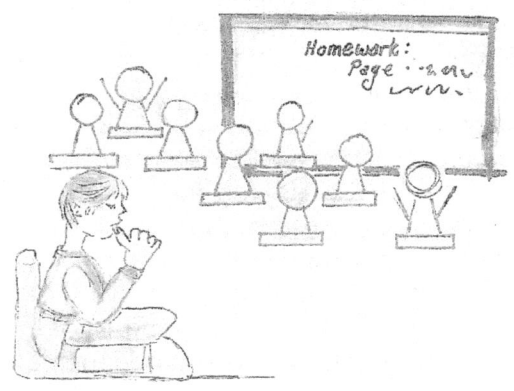

But Ryan is sitting in the back of the room, thumb in his mouth. He is in the "thumb sucking zone", the place where he feels warm and cozy. It is as if he is drifting away on a fluffy white cloud. As a result, Ryan doesn't hear what the teacher is saying. He doesn't hear the questions of the other students and doesn't hear the teacher's careful answers. And, worst of all, he will not know the answers to the quiz questions tomorrow. The comfort of his thumb in his mouth is all he cares about. But, even that comfort will not be able to make up for the embarrassment he will feel when he fails the quiz.

The school day is over at 3:00 p.m. and Ryan is home at last. He is sitting on the sofa in front of the TV. What a relief to sit curled up with his blanket, with his thumb in his mouth,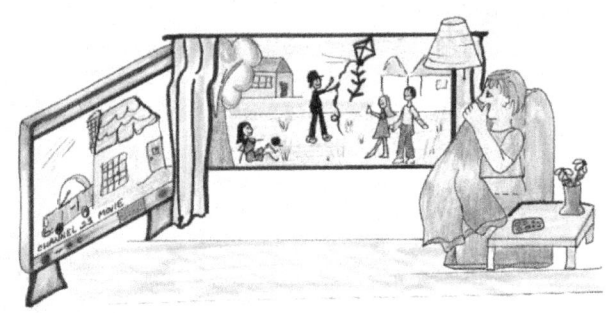
without anyone around to make fun of him. It is a beautiful spring day and most the neighborhood kids are riding their bikes, skateboarding, playing catch and flying kites. Ryan can hear them playing, can hear them laughing and he feels a little tug of regret that he isn't out there with them. But, Ryan would rather stay indoors where he can suck his thumb privately. By the time he thinks he might like to join them after all, it is time to have dinner, and then it is time for bed.

The next day at school Ryan is invited to a sleepover. At first Ryan is excited when he receives the invitation to the sleepover, not just any sleepover, the biggest, best, sleepover of the year. However, after thinking about it, Ryan tells himself he can't go. He is scared to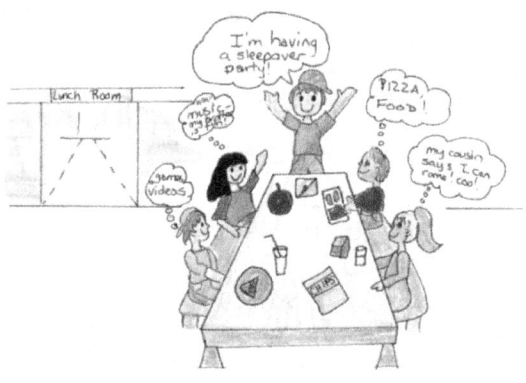
go because he knows that he will suck his thumb. He is afraid of what Stevens, Matt, and P.J. will think when they see him sucking his thumb. He wants to stop, but he knows that he can't do it on his own. He needs someone or something to help him. Unfortunately, he misses out on a very special event because of his thumb sucking.

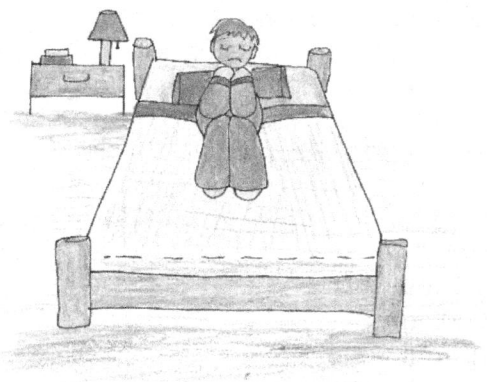

Three days later, Ryan is sitting on his front porch when a few of the neighborhood boys notice him. "Hey, Ryan," Mike yells. "Come over and fly kites with us." "We have an extra kite."

Ryan thinks about joining them, but then politely says, "Maybe later guys. I have stuff I have to do."

But, that is not quite true. Ryan is so hooked on sucking his thumb, the urge to suck takes over no matter what he wants to do. Instead of interacting with friends he prefers to sit idle on the porch zoning out, thumb in his mouth. But even when he is sucking his thumb, he really isn't happy. He thinks to himself, *"Why do I just sit here? Why do I feel left out? Why do I feel angry?"*

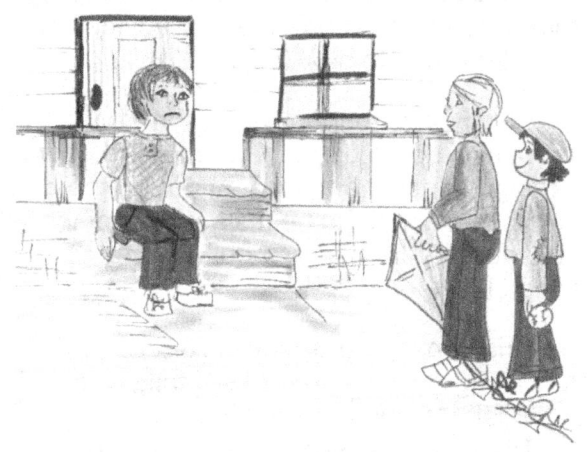

At the beginning of summer, Ryan's mom, dad, sister, Ryan and their dachshund Candy Cane are taking a trip to Grandma and Grandpa's house in Chicago. Everyone is excited about the trip because it has been five long months since their last visit. The trip will take them approximately six hours. The van is loaded with suitcases, bottled water, Gatorade, trail mix, sandwiches, dog treats and Ryan's ipad. Well into the trip Ryan is frustrated because the urge to suck his thumb even gets in the way of playing on his I-pad. His frustration has been building over the past few weeks and he decides that this is the perfect time to say something to his parents. Bravely he says with a note of depression in his voice, "Mom, Dad, I really want to stop sucking my thumb, but today is going to be especially hard because the van is one of the places I most like to suck my thumb." He adds, "I wonder why I get the urge to suck my thumb when I am riding in the van? I start out saying that I won't suck my thumb and then like magic, presto-change-o, my thumb ends up in my mouth."

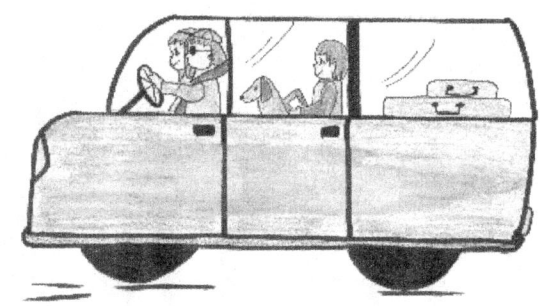

Ryan's family listens patiently. They are not sure they can answer his question but tell him if you want to stop we will help you. His sister never sucked her thumb, but his mother did when she was a little girl. Later, once Ryan and his sister are out of ear shot, Ryan's parents discuss what they might do to help Ryan. They decide to ask the family health care provider for advice. Still, they know that Ryan needs to be ready to stop

Finally determined to do something about his thumb sucking, Ryan speaks up at dinner, "Mom, Dad, I want to talk to you about something. I know I am missing out on too much stuff because I suck my thumb. I missed the best sleepover of the year and I sit around the house when my friends are out playing. I don't want to miss out on anything else!"

The sense of urgency in Ryan's voice is what his parents have been waiting for. They have talked to his doctor, dentist, and orthodontist. All told them Ryan is doing a great deal of damage to his teeth. The orthodontist told them he needs to stop before he gets his braces. If he does not stop sucking his thumb the braces will not work effectively. The three professionals Ryan's parents spoke with all emphasized Ryan needs to be ready to stop before they can do much to help.

Ryan's parents smile and catch Ryan off guard. "This isn't funny," he says. "This is serious."

"We are smiling," his mother tells him with a sparkle in her eyes, "because now that you are ready to stop, we are ready to help you get started."

Finally, Ryan is ready to stop sucking his thumb. He is determined, even eager to get started. He knows that talking to his mom and dad was the first big step. While he feels relief, he is also a little worried about what he will have to do. Still, success is the only option; he knows he is ready and willing to do anything he needs to do. So, now is the time to map out a plan.

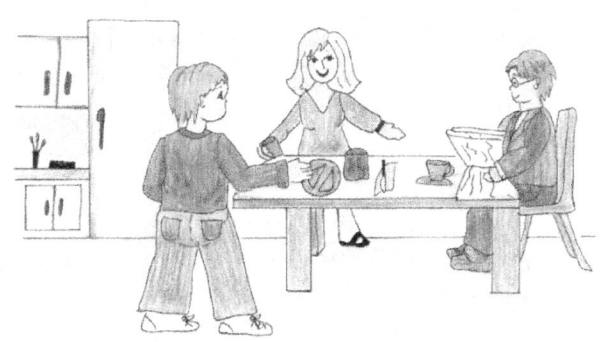

Ryan sits down at the kitchen table with his mother. After consulting professionals, Mom has learned that it is important to ask Ryan a few questions before they get started. She begins the dialogue by asking him, "Ryan, where and when do you like to suck your thumb?"

"Mostly always and anywhere," he says with a resigned smile.

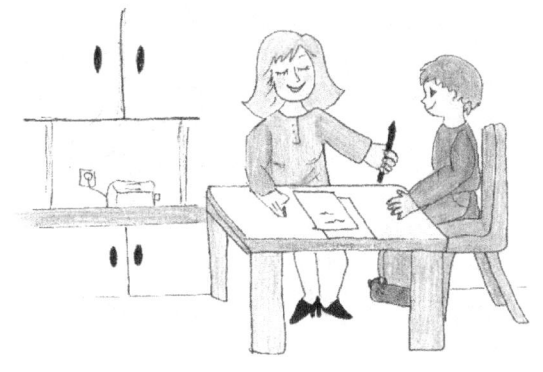

"No," his mother says. "You don't suck when you are eating."

They laugh together, then Ryan starts to give Mom the information they need to get started. "Well", he says, "I do have some favorite times and places."

"Yes," his mother says. "That is what I need to know.

Illustrations by Nancy Ruppert

I have included a few questions you may wish to use to begin your discussion of Ryan's dilemma. You may also wish to add a few questions of your own. Realizing other people/children do or have had to contend with thumb sucking and have managed to change this behavior allows your child to know they are not alone and there is a solution.

Discussion Questions:

- How do you think Ryan felt when the kids on the school bus made fun of him for sucking his thumb and when he missed out on the sleep-over?
- Why do you think Ryan felt the way he did?
- Do you believe Ryan wants to continue feeling this way?
- What do you think Ryan should do to fix the problem?
- Have you ever felt the same way Ryan did in the story?

Reading the story together opens discussion and **Awareness** of thumb sucking which helps determine if your child has the desire to stop. **Education** provides the knowledge to formulate a 'Plan.' When there is a basic understanding of the problem, the foundation on which to build and formulate a 'Plan' to achieve success is in place.

Chapter 4

Prepare for a Thumb Program

Three steps to prepare for a Thumb Program
- Map out a Plan
- Understanding the Goals and Guidelines
- Supplies and Motivational Tools

STEP ONE: Map Out a Plan

Mapping out a plan will better prepare you to help the thumb sucker achieve success. The following facts should be considered if you want a program to be successful. You first need to start with **NORMAL!**

What do I Mean by Normal?
- The child needs to be in good physical, emotional, and psychological health.
- Remember: No disruptions in the home life (divorce, illness, new baby, or moving, etc.)
- Do not start during a holiday.
- Both parents need to agree regarding all facets of the program. If there is a divorce situation and both parents are sharing custody, both parents need to equally participate.

A **POSITIVE** approach is much more fun and generally more successful.

CONFIDENCE - For any program to be successful, confidence in the outcome is imperative.

COOPERATION - Make sure the child is willing to participate in the program. If the child is not ready, no matter what program you choose, NOTHING will work.

Know Your Professionals

A professional possesses valuable expertise to provide help and care. I have listed specific professionals to acquaint you with their specialties. Not every professional will have the knowledge or expertise to help with thumb elimination but, should be able to provide support. After reading this book, you can decide which professional(s) you may want to consult, allowing you to choose wisely.

Find a professional who takes a **positive approach**; someone who works well with children and makes the process fun. This is not the time to scold or punish the child. A system that rewards always works better than a system that punishes.

If you go to a professional for intervention, choose someone with specific expertise to treat thumb sucking. Discuss with your 'professional of choice' their therapeutic philosophy and approach, before you make a commitment. A positive behavior modification approach is recommended as the therapy of choice by most experts (reference Chapter 6). Make sure guidelines are in place before beginning the program. (Example: You need to go 10 days and nights without sucking your thumb before a reward is given). Different therapists deal with relapse differently. Some ask the child to return the reward when they regress back into thumb sucking. Others make the next reward even more attractive. **But, and this is most important, it is best not to reward a flip flopper.** It is best not to reward someone who stops for one day, return to their thumb sucking the next day.

Orofacial Myologist

"An Orofacial Myologist is a professional (core education Speech and Language Pathology or Dental Hygiene). The training in Orofacial Myology involves an individualized program to help individuals retrain these adaptive patterns of muscle function and to create and maintain a healthy oro-facial environment." (IAOM definition) www.iaom.com.
  https://www.google.com/search?q=International+Association+of+Orofacial+Myology&oq=International+Association+of+Orofacial+Myology&aqs=chrome.0

Treatment goals may include the following:
- Thumb/ finger/tongue sucking elimination.
- Prolonged pacifier use elimination.

- Normalize tongue and lip resting postures.
- Establish functional nasal breathing patterns.
- Eliminate improper chewing and swallowing patterns.
- Stabilize the dentition from extraneous oro-facial muscle movement.
- Fingernail, cheek, or lip biting elimination.
- Clenching or grinding of the teeth elimination.

Contact the IAOM directory www.iaom.com for a therapist in your area or contact this author as a resource at www.suburbanmft.com.

Counselor

"Counselors are professionals who offer guidance to individuals, couples, families and groups who are dealing with issues that affect their mental health and well-being. Many counselors approach their work holistically, using a "wellness" model (as opposed to an "illness" one) which highlights and encourages client's strengths." Definition provided by The American School Counselor Association (ASCA.)

https://www.google.com/search?ei=RdWtfDMM65zwKohKTgBg&q=American+school+of+counselor+association&oq=American+school+of+counselor+ass

Psychologist

A psychologist 'is a general practice and health service provider trained in psychology which is the study of the mind and behavior. The discipline embraces all aspects of the human experience — from the functions of the brain to their actions, from child development to care for the aged.' Definition provided by American Psychological Association (APA.)

A psychologist provides a range of psychological diagnosis, assessment, intervention, prevention, health diagnosis, program development and evaluation services with a special focus on the developmental processes of children and youth within the context of schools, families and other systems.

A psychologist is not able to write prescriptions but, may recommend a patient be seen by a fellow psychiatrist to receive medications. Most thumb sucking patterns are habitual; however, there are some thumb sucking patterns that need special evaluation and care before beginning a thumb program. This is when a psychologist should be consulted.

https://www.google.com/search?ei=9u7dWsSXGYPtzgKG7LiABg&q=American+Psychological+Association&oq=American+Psychological+Association&gs_l=p

Psychiatrist

A psychiatrist 'is a medical doctor who specializes in mental health focusing on the diagnosis, treatment and prevention of mental, emotional and behavioral disorders. They often employ individual or group therapy to gain insight into a patient's past and find coping methods to help patients address their own problems.' Definition provided by American Psychiatrist Association (APA.)

Most thumb sucking patterns are habitual; however, there are some thumb sucking patterns that need special evaluation and care before initiating a thumb program. This is when a psychiatrist should be consulted.
https://www.google.com/search?q=Aperican+Psychiatric+Association&oq=Aperican+Psychiatric+Association&aqs=chrome69i57j0l5.9337j0j8&sourceid=ch

Counselor Psychologist Psychiatrist

If it is determined that the possible cause of thumb sucking runs deeper than just a set pattern, NO ACTION or program should be started until you seek advice from one of the professionals mentioned; psychologist, psychiatrist, counselor. If there is a deep underlying cause for the thumb sucking that is not dealt with, the individual may not stop sucking their thumb and or may start to transfer the sucking action to another unwanted pattern, such as wetting the bed.

Speech Pathologist

A speech-language pathologist (SLP) is a professional 'who works to prevent, assess, diagnose, and treat speech, language, social communication, cognitive-communication, and swallowing disorders in children and adults.' Definition provided by the American Speech-Language-Hearing Association (ASHA.)

The speech pathologist in the public schools is not able to treat a thumb sucking problem within the school setting due to state rules and regulations. Most speech and language pathologists will not have the expertise to treat thumb sucking patterns. However, if the speech pathologist has the additional expertise needed to successfully treat a thumb sucking pattern, a COM will be part of their credentials. (If your speech and language pathologist is not able to provide information you

may wish to contact the IAOM directory *www.iaom.com* for a therapist in your area or contact this author as a resource at www.suburbanmft.com
https://www.google.com/search?q=ASHA&oq=ASHA&aqs=chrome.69i57 j69i59j0l4.3104j0j8&sourceid=chrome&es_sm=93&ie=UTF-8

Pediatrician

A pediatrician 'is a doctor with education in the branch of medicine concerned with children, the care and development of children and the prevention and treatment of children's diseases.' Definition provided by the American Academy of Pediatrics (AAP.)

Many pediatricians are unfamiliar with professionals who address thumb sucking patterns. However, more and more pediatricians today are learning about the complexity of thumb sucking and the effects to the patient's overall health and well-being. This child needs to be individually evaluated to determine the length and strength of the pattern and if the pattern needs to be addressed. These pediatricians will have a referral source for you. (If your pediatrician is not able to provide help you may wish to contact the IAOM directory www.iaom.com for a therapist in your area or contact this author as a resource at www.suburbanmft.com
https://www.google.com/search?q=aperican+academy+of+pediatrics&oq =aperican+academy+of+pediatrics&aqs=chrome.69i57j0l5.7615j0j8&sou rceid=ch

Dentist

A dentist 'is a doctor who is trained to care for the teeth and mouth. Dentistry is the science concerned with the development, structure and function of the teeth, jaws, and mouth. The dentist is trained in prevention, diagnosis, and treatment of diseases of the mouth. Dentists' area of care includes teeth, the muscles of the head, neck and jaw, the tongue, salivary glands, the nervous system of the head and neck and other areas. Dentists' training also enables them to recognize situations that warrant referring patients for care by dental specialists or physicians.' Definition provided by American Dental Association (ADA.) The dentist is one of the first professionals who may examine your child. At an early age, the dentist can diagnose any damage the thumb may be doing to the developing dentition.

As a professional, your dentist has the expertise to answer your questions regarding the growth and development of your teeth. Today many D.D.S.'s have embraced the behavior modification approach for sucking pattern elimination over the traditional habit-breaking

appliances. They may have an in-house orofacial myologist or will make a referral to one. (If your dental professional is not able to provide help you may wish to contact the IAOM directory at www.iaom.com for a therapist in your area or contact this author as a resource
https://www.google.com/search?q=American+Dental+Association&oq=American+Dental+Association&aqs=chrome.69i57j0l5.7765j0j8&sourceid=chrome&

Orthodontist

An orthodontist is a doctor who is 'a uniquely qualified specialist able to diagnose, prevent and treat dental and facial irregularities to correctly align teeth and jaws. He specializes in the diagnosis, prevention, and treatment of orthodontic problems, and has completed two to four years of advanced training in an accredited orthodontic residency program.' Definition provided by American Association of Orthodontists (AAO.)

Ask your orthodontist about thumb sucking complications and elimination. Chapter 6, 'The Professional Connection', highlights this pertinent information.

Orthodontists that are aware of behavior modification techniques are embracing this approach and may have an in-house orofacial myologist or will make a referral to one. If your orthodontist is not able to provide help you may wish to contact the IAOM directory www.iaom.com for a therapist in your area.

Even when professionals are involved, it is equally important all family members also get involved, including siblings. This needs to be a 'team effort.' Everyone needs to encourage, not criticize. Teasing will only prevent success. In my experience, the therapist needs to make sure that siblings don't feel left out when they see the amount of attention being given to the thumb sucking child. Ask siblings to help. Becoming involved prevents siblings from feeling left out. Make teachers and grandparents aware of the intervention program too. The individual trying to stop thumb sucking will appreciate all encouragement.

STEP TWO: Understanding the Goals and Guidelines
This Author's Tried and True Goals and Guidelines

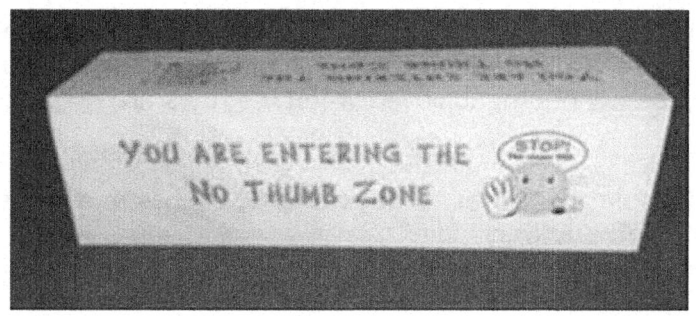

Goal 1: The child will be able to complete 10 days and nights in a row with no thumb sucking

Upon completion of this first goal, acknowledge this successful accomplishment with a motivational reward. I like this to be fun, so I tell the child, "Mom and Dad do not know they will be buying you a present," (then I laugh.) The child gets a big kick out of this statement. I explain to the child, "The present is a way for your parents to express how proud they are in what you have achieved thus far." The present should not be expensive, not exceed $10.00 to $15.00. This should not be considered a bribe. This is a way parents can acknowledge how proud they are of their child in achieving this accomplishment. You want your child to succeed.

Do not reward a flip-flopper

A flip-flopper is a child, whom after receiving a present, resumes sucking their thumb. If the child, after receiving their present, returns to sucking their thumb, they will have to give the present back to the gift giver until they complete another 10 days and nights in a row with no thumb sucking. This needs to be made clear when the rules are presented.

Caution: Thumb suckers have been known to quit sucking within the first couple of days on the program. When this happens, the child usually becomes overconfident deciding, "This is so easy. I no longer need to do some of the tasks required." That is when the decision to change or eliminate some of the rules occurs. In my experience, not following the rules leads to relapse. It takes at least a month for a pattern to weaken, diminishing the urge to suck.

Caution: Parents can be just as bad. Many parents when their child does well quickly, can become equally overconfident and stop following the program procedures. That is when I tell the child, "We are all equal here and if I find out Mom and Dad are not following the rules, I (the therapist) will reprimand them right in front of you." (Kids love this). Success will not be achieved when the rules are not followed by everyone.

Goal 2: Complete another 10 days and 10 nights in a row with no thumb sucking
Receive a second motivational reward.

Goal 3: The program is completed and successful when the child has not sucked their thumb day or night consecutively for a month

CELEBRATE! I (the therapist) always provide my thumb graduates with a thumb certificate to acknowledge their achievement of thumb sucking elimination. Parents can celebrate with their child by doing a favorite activity in acknowledgement of how proud they are of their child's success.

The One Month Rule
In my experience, when treating thumb sucking, the usual scenario is that thumb sucking stops within one to three days. However, even if the child stops immediately, **the program must continue for one full month.** It takes at least one month to fully address the sucking pattern; reduce the urge to suck, learn and implement the skills needed to control the urge to suck, and build confidence and independence from their thumb. **There are no short cuts.**

Purpose
- It takes approximately a month to establish a new pattern.
- It takes a month to stabilize the new pattern. Within that month, the child will experience an array of feelings: highs and lows, good days and bad, calm and stressful days. They need to navigate these days without reverting to the coping mechanism of sucking their thumb.
- The child needs to recognize trigger times and then utilize coping skills the therapist has introduced.
- In my experience when the child spontaneously tells me, "I never think about my thumb anymore," and/or, "I do not have the urge to suck my thumb anymore," then I know this child is ready to be dismissed from therapy. Their positive, spontaneous statements illustrate the confidence this child has achieved and confirms a

solid foundation has been established to maintain this successful non-sucking pattern on their own. The child is ready to graduate.

A Lay Person (Non-Professional) Home Program

If a parent is attempting to do this program at home without a therapist's expertise, the parent needs to make sure to read the _Two Thumbs Up_ book entirely. You need to have a thorough understanding of the thumb sucking pattern. You need to understand what your child is going through physically, emotionally, and chemically. (A detailed explanation provided in Chapter 6)

- The parent and child both need to understand and follow all rules of the program.
- The program needs to be fun, exciting and positive.
- The parents and the entire family need to be supportive and compassionate. Remember, if this were a cigarette habit you would not expect the smoker to just put the cigarette down and stop without having frequent urges to smoke.

A Trained Professional - Orofacial Myologist

A trained orofacial myologist has the expertise to evaluate each step, identify triggers causing pitfalls and deal with them. Even though parents are following the program twenty-four hours a day, a trained therapist, meeting with the child, will recognize triggers and pitfalls not noticed by the parents. For this reason, an orofacial myologist schedules weekly meetings as part of the program. Sometimes working with someone outside the family circle is a better choice.

Rules Must Be Followed

- Bed must be at a decent hour even on weekends. Weekend bedtime may be extended, but no more than 1 ½ hours. The longer the child stays up, the more exhausted they become and the less control they have subconsciously.
- The child must sleep in their own bed the first 10 nights.
- There should be no sleepovers the first 10 nights. The chances of obtaining a good night's sleep and eating correctly are doubtful during a sleepover. This program requires both, so I would discourage any sleepover during this time.
- They should have no refined sugar, heavy foods, cereal, soda pop, ice cream, etc. 1 ½ hours before bed. Consuming heavy foods and or refined sugar may sabotage the success of the program. Children like to have sugar before bed, however, the effects of sugar can be counter-productive. Sugar can be a stimulant hyping

the child up before bed, which is what we do not want to happen. At bedtime we want our thumb sucker to be calm and relaxed. Instead, if they want a snack at bedtime make it something natural. (Example, a piece of fresh fruit). Also, sugar consumption increases the urge to urinate disrupting the sleep pattern. We want our thumb sucker to sleep throughout the night. If the child wakes up in the middle of the night and needs to go to the bathroom, chances are when they return to bed, they will put their thumb in their mouth to fall back to sleep out of habit.

Facts About Sugar - Statistics*
- Sugar is America's number one food additive.
- The American Heart Association recommends we consume less than ten teaspoons of sugar a day. The average child consumes 32 teaspoons a day.
- There are connections of eating more sugar with high blood pressure, blood sugar concerns, mood instabilities, acne, headaches, fatigue, hyperactivity, aching joints, and tooth decay.
- Sugar also robs the body of vitamins and minerals. Refined sugar not only contains no nutrients, for the sugar to be metabolized it must draw on the body's reserve of vitamins and minerals.
    *Dr. Meaghan Kirschling, DC, APRN, RN, MS
    http://beyondthebasicshealthacademy.com/children-sugar-staggering-statistics/

The Sugar Habit - Effects on The Body
- Sugar can cause a rapid rise in adrenaline, hyperactivity, anxiety, difficulty concentrating, and crankiness in children.
- Sugar can cause your saliva to become acidic, tooth decay, and periodontal disease.
- Sugar may worsen the symptoms of children with attention deficit hyperactivity disorder (ADHD).
- Sugar increases the activity of the adrenal glands forcing them to secrete more adrenaline into the body.
- Refined sugars form carbohydrates & are processed quickly in your body.
- Sugar causes the body to release more of the nutrients and vitamins it already has through urination therefore, will increase the frequency of urination.

References:
Appleton, Nancy PhD (1988) "Lick The Sugar Habit: Sugar Addiction Upsets Your Whole Body Chemistry." Penguin Publishing Group.
https://articles.mercola.com/sugar-addiction.aspx

Prinz, Robert, et al. (1980) "Dietary Correlates of Hyperactive Behavior in Children." Journal of Consulting and Clinical Psychology, vol. 48, no. 6, pp. 760–769.

Jones, T W, et al. (1995) "Enhanced Adrenomedullary Response and Increased Susceptibility to Neuroglycopenia: Mechanisms Underlying the Adverse Effects of Sugar Ingestion in Healthy Children." The Journal of Pediatrics, vol. 126, no. 2, pp. 171–177.

https://www.nytimes.com/1995/03/15/us/study-sees-a- sugar-adrenaline-link-in-children.html

https://www.livestrong.com/article/553512-does-a-lot-of-sugar-in-your-diet-make-you-pee-more/

https://www.livestrong.com/article/376125-high-sugar-consumption-symptoms

STEP THREE: Supplies and Motivational Tools
After decades of addressing this multi-faceted complex pattern, I have refined, changed, and added tools that motivate and simplify the therapeutic process. In my experience, one way to simplify and help busy parents is to provide options. The first option is a 'Thumb Kit', which includes all necessary materials. Not all therapists provide a 'Thumb Kit' option. The second option is a check list of necessary materials the parent will need to purchase. Discuss with your therapist of choice their therapeutic process. Below I've listed all materials utilized in my treatment program, along with option one and option two for your perusal.

Thumb Kit
In my experience, many working parents have difficulty finding extra time in their already busy schedules to buy all necessary procedure materials. Therefore, in my practice I provided parents two options. A Thumb Kit', which includes all necessary materials. (Not all therapists provide a 'Thumb Kit' option). The second option is a check list of necessary materials the parent will need to purchase.

Materials in my Thumb Kit
- Detailed directions and procedures
- Wooden spoon-to make Spoon Person
- Materials to embellish Spoon Person
- Stickers
- Neon Band-Aids
- Ten-day reward medallion
- Motivational cards and corresponding theme items
- Sample thumb chart
- Sample Thumb Certificate

Sample notes to be placed on bed ½ hour before bed

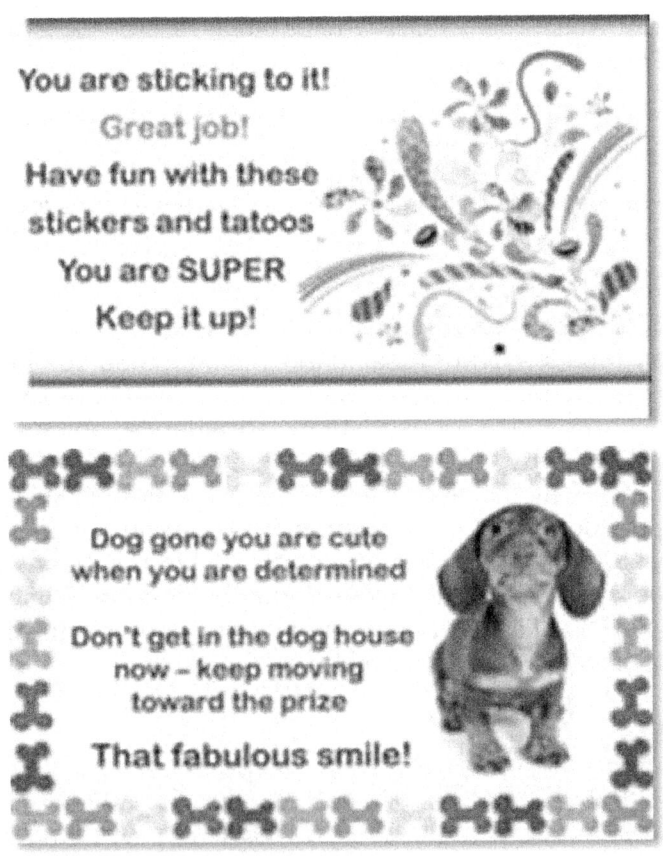

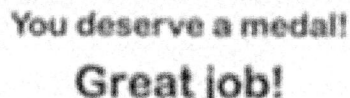

You deserve a medal!
Great job!
Tomorrow
ten days and nights
without sucking your thumb

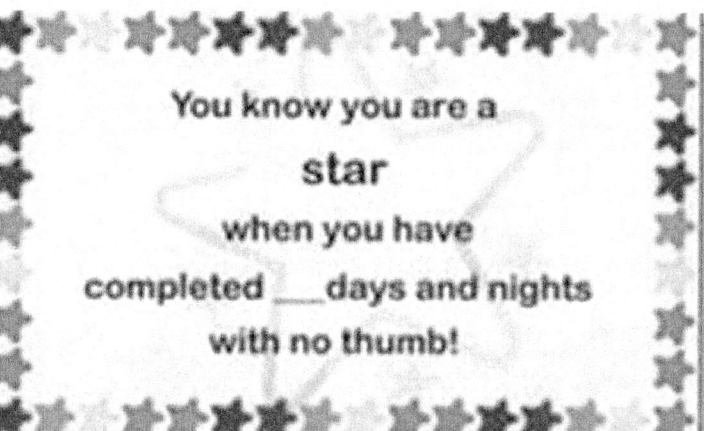

You know you are a
star
when you have
completed ___ days and nights
with no thumb!

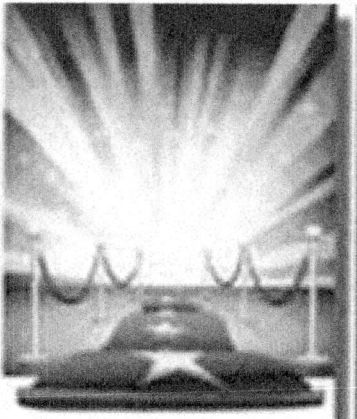

Write your own ticket to success. You have gone ___ days and nights with no thumb.

Corresponding theme items to accompany each note

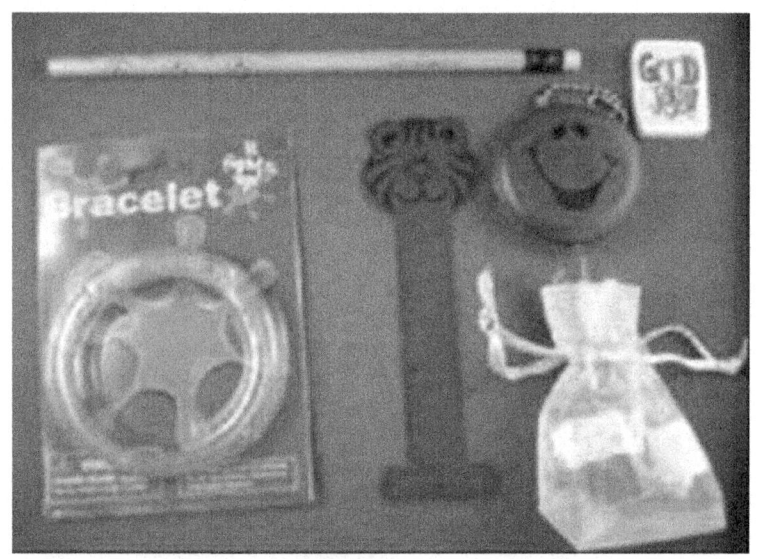

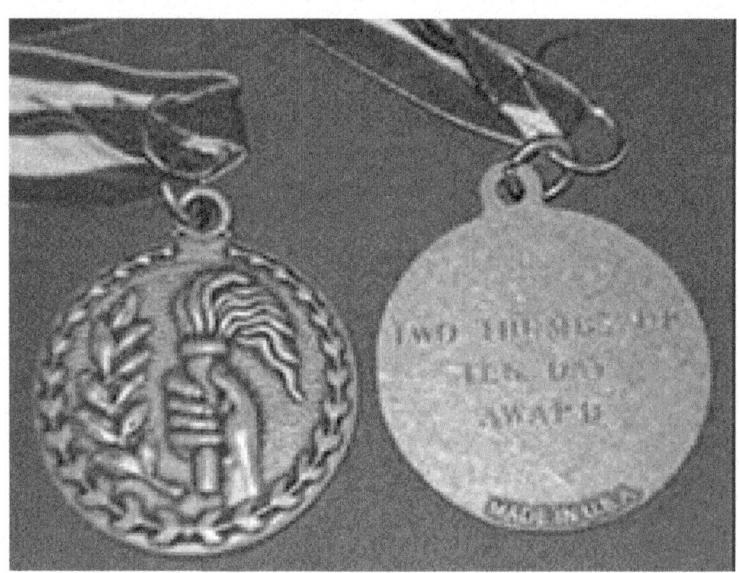

Conscious awareness items

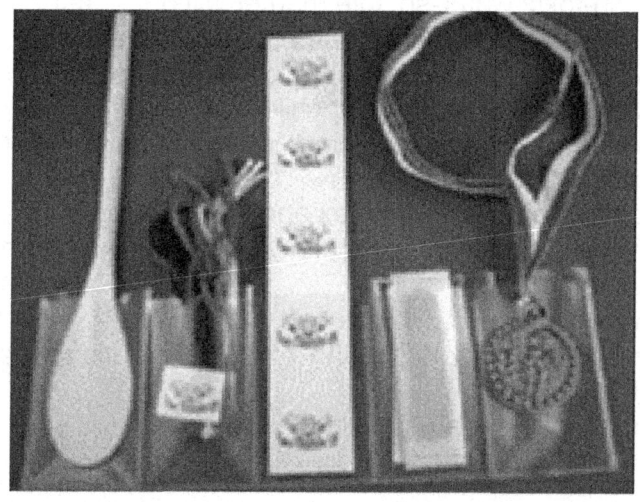

Spoon & accessories to make Spoon Person Face

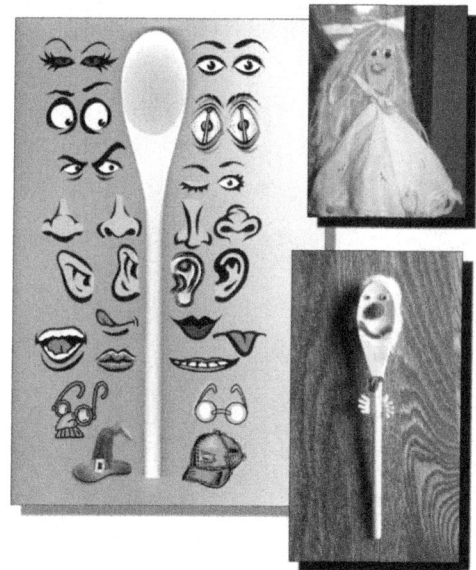

Here is a sample of 'Spoon People' my thumb patients made while going through the thumb program. "I think they did a great job! What do you think"?

Option Two - Parents Purchase Materials
Materials needed:
- Ace-Bandage or non-stretch cloth gauze
- Cloth adhesive tape (ex. surgical tape, athletic tape (must use cloth tape or non-toxic water-soluble marker will not adhere)
- 3 safety pins or may use cloth tape to secure bandage or gauze
- Water-soluble non-toxic markers (only use non-toxic markers, other markers could make your child sick)
- Construction paper, poster board, or computer paper to make a thumb chart
- Shoe box to create a thumb box and store all items
- Neon colored Band-Aids or Birdie Digit Tape for emergencies
- Motivational stickers
- Items to place on pillow before bed
- Wooden spoon to make Spoon Person (2 spoons to make Spoon People if switch-hitter)
- Books, magazines, games, etc.

Chapter 5

Sample Step by Step Thumb Program

This sample step by step Thumb Program represents successful therapeutic **Treatment** this therapist has embraced for decades. This sample maps out a therapeutic journey: from addressing the 'Trigger' causing the thumb sucking 'Call to Action,' to Step by Step procedures and objectives. Various helpful hints and potential pitfalls to avoid are also highlighted. Upon completion of this program ideas to acknowledge your child's Success is presented.

First Address the 'Trigger'
Most thumb suckers have a favorite blanket, pillow, or stuffed animal they love to hold and or carry around while sucking their thumb. This object is a '**call to action**' whispering in their ear, "It is time to start sucking." For that reason, the first step is to address this favorite article we call the '**trigger.**'

A Trigger is a Cue a Call to Action
The trigger can be **physical.** An example of this might be a pillow, blanket, stuffed animal, clothing, hair, etc. A trigger can also be **emotional**. An example might be the urge to suck when feeling tired, bored, sad, upset, needing comfort, thus, sucking becomes a pain reliever, calms and soothes and a built-in pacifier. We at this time will be addressing the physical trigger.
This is a must. Send the trigger on vacation. Place the blanket, stuffed animal, doll, etc., (whatever you perceive to be the trigger) on the highest shelf in a closet. The thumb sucker will know where the article is, however, will not be able to hold it. If the child continues to hold the article, the urge to suck the thumb will not diminish.

Be Prepared. This is probably the toughest thing for the child to do. Explain to the child this article needs to go on vacation and will be returned upon completion of the program. When the child makes the decision to allow the item to go on vacation, this action becomes a positive. I think we all can agree a vacation is a positive. The parent and child will pick a closet and place the 'trigger' on the highest shelf in that closet (the vacation spot). The child will know where the article is and can go to the closet and check for reassurance that it is still there, however, will not be able to take it down and hold it during weak moments. Sending the article on vacation shows the willingness to try and is the first positive step in a successful program.

Beware of Idle Time

Watching TV and riding in a car are idle-times, often danger zones, times when that sneaky thumb may find its way into the child's mouth. If this is problematic, the best thing to do is to try to keep the hands away from the mouth. During idle-time the thumb will seem to have a mind of its own and sneak into the mouth before the child becomes aware that the thumb has reached its target. Then it is **too late!**

Activities, Books, Magazines, Games - The 20 Minute Pass
Purpose:

Activities allow the child to redirect their focus. Buy and retain a host of books, magazines, games (items of child's interest) available to the child when they have the urge to suck. You do not want to use items they already have. The items need to be unfamiliar and new to them, making the item they choose for the 20-Minute Pass exciting and distracting. When the child has the urge to thumb suck, provide one of these items/activities. If the child learns to keep busy for a period of at least twenty minutes, the urge usually passes. It is like being on a diet; if the image of chocolate cake enters the mind, the savvy dieter has something healthier nearby to munch on which satisfies the craving to eat something or finds an activity to keep their mind occupied. In other word, avoid temptation and idle-time. Do not leave these items laying around before or following the 20-Minute Pass.

Procedure:

When the child has the urge to suck, that is when the parent will provide one of these items/activities. The parent only provides the item when the urge to suck needs to be deterred.

Object - Items to Hold
Purpose:
    One successful way to help keep the thumb out of the mouth during idle-time is to have the child hold an object in the thumb sucking hand. (Remember, the closer the hand is to the mouth the easier it is for the thumb to sneak in unaware to the thumb sucker until it is too late.) Holding an object not only helps to keep the hand/thumb away from the face but also helps the child become aware when the hand moves up toward the face getting too close to the mouth. By creating a spoon person, the child utilizes their creativity and imagination, as well as, having fun preparing to begin their program (positive actions- positive thinking).

Procedure:
    Have the child draw or paint a face, hair and ears if they wish, on the spoon to create the '**Spoon Person**'. Suggest to the child they might name the spoon (to personalize it). Once the spoon person has been created the child will hold the spoon during idle-times, as a special friend, that will help to remind them to keep their hand away from their face. The 'Spoon Person' should be held during idle times such as; T.V. time, listening to a story and can easily accompany the child in the car. Remember to bring the spoon person to the next therapy appointment for 'show and tell.'

Make a Thumb Box
Purpose & Procedure:
    Give the child an old shoe box and tell them they can decorate this box transforming it from a shoe box into their 'Thumb Box.'
This is done for the following reasons...
- Creativity: Allows the child to be creative while doing something positive with their idle-time. Use the Thumb Box to hold tape, pins, Ace-Bandage or gauze, notes, chart and surprises already received from the bedtime pillow. (Chart and surprises on bedtime pillow will be discussed later in this chapter). Bring the box with its contents to the next appointment for 'show and tell'.
- Organized: Keeping everything in the box helps to stay organized and prepared for bedtime. There is nothing worse than not knowing where the child's materials are when needed. We do not want the routine to be altered, for example, the dog ran off with the ace bandage or gauze, no one can find it and it is past the child's bedtime. The goal is to have bedtime calm and organized, not chaotic and disruptive.

- Proud: During the next appointment the child will show the therapist their Spoon Person and everything they received on their pillow along with their marked chart. The therapist and child discuss how the child is doing, ask the child how they are feeling, and ask if anyone has questions. The therapist may then want to take the child's picture with their thumb chart and spoon person acknowledging the child's achievement to this point.

Make a Thumb Chart
Purpose:
Have the child create a Thumb Chart to track their progress. Creating their own chart, writing a saying about the thumb, drawing a picture about the thumb, utilizing their favorite stickers, all are very positive steps in the program.

Procedure:
Take a piece of computer paper or construction paper and make a Thumb Chart. On the top half of the paper the child can draw a picture, trace their thumb, write a funny saying about the thumb etc. On the bottom half of the chart divide it into day - night and, if needed, school.

Sample Thumb Chart

	Mon	*Tues*	*Wed*	*Thurs*	*Fri*	*Sat*	*Sun*
Day							
School							
Night							

If the child switches from right thumb to left thumb, having no thumb preference, I call them a 'Switch Hitter.' Then I have the child do (right-day, school, night) and (left-day, school, night.) This makes it is easier to keep track of how well each thumb is doing.

Sample Thumb Chart for Switch Hitter

Right Thumb	Mon	Tues	Wed	Thurs	Fri	Sat	Sun
Day							
School							
Night							

Left Thumb	Mon	Tues	Wed	Thurs	Fri	Sat	Sun
Day							
School							
Night							

Marking the Chart
Purpose:

    Daytime is from the time the child gets out of bed to the time the child gets back into bed. Place the star on chart right before bed acknowledging how the child did during the day.

    School is from the time the child leaves for school to the time the child returns home from school. Place the star on the chart when the child gets home from school. If your child does not thumb suck at school, 'school' does not have to be listed on their chart.

    Nighttime is from the time the child gets into bed until they get out of bed. Place a star on the chart when your child gets out of bed.

    Naps: If your child still takes a nap, that is considered night time (even if it is light outside).

Procedure:

    People generally associate stars with a positive symbol. Using stars on the chart makes the procedure fun. The parent can buy stars to be placed on the chart each day. (Follow marking the chart directions.) The second option is for the child to draw a star on their chart.

Follow marking the chart directions
- A whole star is marked on their chart if no sucking occurred.
- A ½ star is marked on their chart if they did suck but followed the rules. 'Trying' is the key word. It is the parent's job to be the cheerleader providing positive comments and motivation. (After placing the half star on the chart, write the determined reason why they sucked their thumb next to the half star. Example: took tape off, forgot to put tape on, stayed up past bedtime, ate refined sugar or heavy foods before bed, was punished and still upset when went to bed.)

Daytime Agenda
All Day Cloth Adhesive Tape (1 long piece worn all day)
The face is a danger zone. The thumb can be very sneaky, always wanting to enter the mouth. Many thumb suckers like to have their hands close to or on their face. This is a NO, NO! When their hands are near or on the face, it becomes too easy for the thumb to slip into the mouth before the child can stop it. Therefore, the child needs to have tools and reminders to keep hands away from their face until this pattern changes.

Purpose:
The cloth adhesive tape is the tape of choice because it allows the non-toxic, water-soluble marker to adhere, while a rubber textured tape (like a Band-Aid) will not adhere and the marker will slide right off. The cloth adhesive tape and bright colored, non-toxic marker provide a way to remind the child to keep their hands away from their face (conscious awareness.)

Procedure:
Take one long piece of cloth adhesive tape and wrap the nail and that part of the thumb circling the thumb a couple of times so the tape will adhere to the skin and adhere to the adhesive tape. (Do not cover the knuckle. The thumb needs to be able to bend and not feel as if it is being restrained.) **In emergencies** when the tape is not readily available, use bright neon Band-Aids (discussed later in this chapter). **Caution:** Do not allow child to discontinue tape or Band-Aid on their own. If the tape is discontinued too soon, the urge to suck the thumb will not have had time to weaken. When the thumb sucking action remains strong, the thumb remains in control instead of the child being in control.

Water Soluble Non-Toxic Marker
Purpose:
    The bright, water-soluble, non-toxic marker provides a visual aid bringing it to your child's attention if the thumb tries to sneak up to and into the mouth. If your child sucks their thumb, the water-soluble, non-toxic marker will smear or be gone, telling everyone sucking occurred. **Only Use Water Soluble, Non-toxic markers!** (Other markers could make your child sick.)

Procedure:
    Draw a star, heart or smiley face, etc. on the tape over the nail. Change the color of the non-toxic, water-soluble marker every time you transition from daytime, to nighttime, to school time. Variety will help the child to consciously maintain an awareness if the thumb moves up toward the mouth. Most kids have a favorite color and will have the tendency to want to use that color all the time. I do not recommend the use of the same color non-toxic, water-soluble marker all the time. The too familiar color becomes boring, routine, invisible, and then soon the thumb is again sneaking into the mouth.

Neon Colored Band-Aid or Birdie Digit Tape
Use for emergency purposes only!
Purpose and Procedure:
- At school, if the child's tape gets wet or falls off, a neon Band-Aid or Birdie Digit Tape can be substituted until they return home to replace the Band-Aid or Birdie Digit Tape with new cloth tape and water soluble, non-toxic marker.
- After swimming the Band-Aid or Birdie Digit Tape needs to be used until the child returns home to replace the Band-Aid or Birdie Digit Tape with cloth tape and water-soluble, non-toxic marker.
- If the parent needs to unexpectedly run errands with their child and the cloth tape is not on the child's thumb, the Band-Aid or Birdie Digit Tape allows the parent to improvise, utilizing the Band-Aid or Birdie Digit Tape until they return home and re-tape the thumb with cloth tape. Place the Band-Aid or Birdie Digit Tape over the nail, circling the thumb, the same as you do the cloth adhesive tape.
- Birdie Digit Tape - https://www.birdiesmart.com/shop/digit

School - Inform the Teacher
Purpose and Procedure
- Send a note to the teacher informing her your child is on a thumb sucking elimination program.

- Request the teacher inform you (the parent) if the thumb goes in the child's mouth while at school. Remember the thumb can be Sneaky and the child may not consciously be aware their thumb went into their mouth.
- **Procedure** - Ask the teacher to help at school. Explain if the child gets their hands dirty or wet and the tape they wore to school needs to be replaced, a neon Band-Aid or Birdie Digit Tape can be substituted until they return home to place new cloth adhesive tape and non-toxic marker on. Ask the teacher if she would keep the neon Band-Aids in her desk drawer just in case the need arises. Then provide the child a neon Band-Aid to replace the soiled one.

NOTE:
- The child may be apprehensive about wearing the tape at school. Advise them, if anyone asks, just say, "Mom put it on me." That usually satisfies the questions.
- If your child likes to suck their thumb when they are being read to and story time is a routine at school, you may wish to ask the teacher if you (mom) and your child may speak to the class (with your child's permission). The parent and child can explain the Spoon Person and why it is being held. Express your appreciation to them for helping your child in his thumb sucking elimination program. Once the children are included, they usually become very helpful, preventing ridicule, teasing, and bullying.

Nighttime Materials Needed
- Elastic bandage or non-stretch gauze (If the child is a switch-hitter, you will need to use 2 elastic bandages or gauze.)
- 3 safety pins (The prongs that come with elastic bandages are too sharp and are not recommended. You will have to use 6 safety pins if your child is a switch-hitter.)
- Cloth adhesive tape
- Water-soluble, non-toxic marker

Nighttime - 1 Hour Before Bed
Cloth Adhesive Tape & Non-Toxic Marker
Purpose:
    The adhesive tape and non-toxic marker is to alert the parent and child if thumb sucking occurs while asleep. Make sure the parent only uses cloth adhesive tape because tape that feels like a Band-Aid will not retain the marker and the marker will slide off. If the thumb

goes in the mouth and gets wet from saliva, the marker will be smeared or gone monitoring and verifying results. This technique not only verifies results it prevents potential denial and excuses. Using the tape and marker also allows the parents the benefit of getting a good night sleep and still have an accurate account of thumb or no thumb sucking while their child is in bed or asleep. **Remind your child they cannot take the tape off themselves.** This deters conflicts and denial if thumb sucking occurred. **Caution:** Some kids sweat and cover their head with their blanket at night. If the marker smears, check face and neck for marker. If the marker smears from sweating, it will be visible at place of contact.

Procedure:
- The thumb sucking child should have pajamas on and teeth brushed, ready for bed.
- Take two long pieces of cloth adhesive tape and wrap one long, single piece of tape over the nail in a circular motion covering the nail and the back of the thumb overlapping the tape on itself. Do the same above the thumb joint. Do not cover the knuckle. The thumb needs to be able to bend. Then, take a water-soluble, non-toxic marker and draw a star, a heart, smiley face or picture of your choice on the tape over the nail. Let the marker dry.
- *Remember to use a water-soluble, non-toxic marker. This is imperative.

½ Hour Before Bed
Something Funny Placed on Pillow

Purpose and Procedure:
- Making bedtime a pleasant and positive event will make it easier for the child to maintain a positive attitude, as well as, feel less anxious at bedtime. One way to do this is to provide a note of encouragement, a small reward, a funny note, a funny saying, etc., and gear the item to your thumb sucker. Parents, this is the time for your 'funny side' to come out.
- The child should stay out of their bedroom ½ hour before bed.
- Parents or siblings will make something funny to be placed on pillow. Several funny notes or sayings about the thumb can be made ahead of time and kept out of sight, then each night place one on the child's pillow. Remember, some nights parents are rushed or extremely tired. If the notes are made ahead of time, the parent will always be prepared.

- A parent or sibling will sneak into the child's bedroom and place a note and little surprise on pillow. When the child goes to bed that night, the note will be waiting for them to read, enjoy, and remind them not to suck their thumb. Providing something on the pillow is extremely important. This reduces their anxiety regarding going to bed with no thumb. They are curious to find out what is on the pillow making it fun, not anxious to go to bed. (Samples of notes and items that can be placed on the pillow are displayed in the all-inclusive Thumb Kit area.)
- Don't forget to have the child tell a parent, "I am not going to suck my thumb." Verbally saying this sentence is fun, helps to reinforce and transfer this positive thought into the child's sub-conscience.
- Parents, **please** do not discontinue or forget this step. In my experience, when the child stops thumb sucking quickly, the parent thinks this step is not necessary. BIG MISTAKE! Each step in this program has a purpose and needs to be followed to the letter to achieve and stabilize successful thumb sucking elimination. Positive Reinforcement.

Right Before Bedtime
Elastic Bandage or Non-Stretch Gauze
Purpose:

If the child bends their elbow to suck their thumb, the elastic bandage or gauze will tighten making the child aware they are sucking the thumb and pull it out of their mouth. I am sure you have had your arm or foot fall asleep before. We all do the same thing. We need to shake our arm or stomp our foot to make that funny feeling go away. The same premise applies here; child will straighten their arm when the wrap tightens.

Procedure:

Wrap the naked arm with an elastic bandage from ½ inch below the shoulder to ½ inch above the wrist, **firmly, but not too tight**. Make sure the arm is straight when wrapping. Once wrapped, bend the child's arm to make sure the elbow remains covered and the elastic bandage does not split at the elbow. Secure with 3 safety pins. Then put the pajama top back on. Once the child has completed 10 nights in a row with no thumb sucking, the elastic bandage or gauze can be eliminated, but not before.

Inform your child of the consequences if they return to thumb sucking. If they start sucking their thumb again they will have to go back to using the elastic bandage and or gauze for another consecutive 10 days and nights. Remember the longer the child consistently goes without the thumb the more the urge to suck diminishes and the weaker the set pattern becomes.

Option: Non-Stretch Gauze
Wrap the arm from 3 inches below the elbow to 3 inches above the elbow, overlapping the gauze. If the elbow bends the gauze will tighten. Before the parent secures the gauze with tape or safety pins (your option), bend the child's elbow to make sure the elbow is not exposed when bent. Secure with safety pins (or tape) in three areas to keep in place. **Caution:** If the parent has never used an elastic bandage or non-stretch gauze, it is better to wrap the arm a little loose than too tight. If too tight, the hand, fingers, or top of hand will begin to swell.

The parents should go in ½ hour to 1 hour after your child goes to bed to check on their hand to make sure it is not swelling. In most cases, your child will be able to tell you if it is too-tight when you are wrapping the arm.

Three Regular Size Safety Pins
Purpose:
Secure the elastic bandage or non-stretch gauze in 3 places with a safety pin to prevent the elastic bandage from slipping down the arm or falling off. I recommend using the safety pins instead of the prongs that come with elastic bandage to avoid any possible injury of being poked.

Procedure:
Once you have wrapped the arm with the elastic bandage or gauze you will secure it by placing one safety pin ½ inch below the shoulder, the second safety pin just below the elbow (so the elbow can still bend) and secure the third safety pin ½ inch above the wrist.

Nighttime - Parents Go the Extra Mile
Sucking the thumb at bedtime and while asleep may need a little more attention. The child who sucks their thumb at bedtime feels they cannot get to sleep without sucking. If the child is extremely anxious the parents need to go the extra mile. Tell the child, "I will sit in your bedroom until you fall asleep". Just knowing a parent is in their room helps the child to relax. Usually the child will fall asleep within a half hour. Once your child receives their first whole star each night gets easier. As your child earns a couple of stars, your child's

confidence will grow stronger and the parent will no longer need to sit in their child's bedroom. **Caution:** Do not let 'going the extra mile' become a habit. Once the child completes the first or second night with no thumb sucking, a parent should not have to sit in the room. The key word is 'Positive.' Help your child stay positive, encourage success, and be your child's cheerleader.

Parental Morning Checks

Parental morning checks involve the parents checking to see if the marker is intact when the child wakes. Did the marker remain intact or was the marker smeared or gone? If the marker is intact, not smeared or gone the child did not suck their thumb that night. **Praise your child.**

If the marker is smeared or gone sucking the thumb occurred. If the child sucked their thumb while asleep, they may be disappointed and upset. This is when the parent needs to express **understanding and encouragement** Tell your child, "We will figure out why you sucked your thumb". Remind your child, "This is a learning experience for the entire family and you will do better tonight". Have your child mark their chart with the appropriate star illustrating how they did that night. Remember: a whole star means no thumb sucking and a half star means they sucked but received a half star for trying.

Positive Environment & Discovery

If there is a thumb sucking incident there are two very important points to remember. First, it is important to maintain a **positive environment**. Negativity does not promote a positive environment or the desire to succeed. **Discovery** is equally important. Discover what may have triggered this thumb sucking incident. Asking questions helps us to identify the trigger. Remember the trigger may be a physical object or a response to an emotional feeling. Once the trigger is identified and discussion ensued, skills can be learned deterring unwanted repetitive actions. **Keep it positive - Skills can be learned.**

Discovery Questions
- Ask what happened. Did the child have a bad day at school, get into a fight with their best friend, upset about something, or disciplined for something?
- Did the child and parent follow the directions to the letter?
- Did the child keep their tape on or remove it after the parents left the bedroom?

- What was the child's attitude at bedtime, anxious, uncooperative?
- Was your child not feeling well or have a fever?
- Did the child eat something they were not supposed to before bed?

If the child sucked their thumb, the child needs to call or text the therapist to discuss what happened. We need to try and figure out what triggered the sucking. We do not want to wait until the next appointment. Anxiety can set in and multiply causing doubt and disappointment which will jeopardize the program if not addressed right away. The therapist will be able to ask the child questions to determine what triggered the thumb sucking and council the child and parent how to address the trigger. The therapist is there to analyze, advise, encourage, and provide parents and child guidance and support. The therapist needs to remember parents can become as discouraged, as their child. Positive reinforcement is equally important for child and parent. "We will have success if we stay positive. We can do this together."

After the child has completed 10 consecutive days and nights with no thumb sucking, the therapist will eliminate the elastic bandage or non-stretch gauze. The child will continue to use only the adhesive tape for the next 10 consecutive days and nights. Kids love when the Elastic bandage or gauze is eliminated from the program.

A Reward System - Motivation to Succeed
Purpose:
You want your child motivated to succeed. I have found that a reward system is an excellent motivator. When the child completes the first 10 days and nights in a row with no thumb sucking the child receives a **present** (reward) from the parents. The therapist can explain the present is a way for the parents to express how proud they are of their child for not sucking their thumb.

Procedure:
When the child completes 10 days and nights in a row with no thumb sucking I say to the child, "You will receive a present from your parents for successfully completing 10 days and nights with no thumb sucking". I then explain with laughter, "Mom and Dad did not know they would be giving you a present. Usually, the child gets a big kick out of this statement.

If the parent buys a present instead of making one, the present should not be expensive or exceed $10.00 to $15.00. This present is a reward not a bribe. Whatever the present is make sure your child understands how proud you are of them in achieving this accomplishment. Make it a **PARTY**.

Remember do not reward a flip flopper. If the child, after receiving their present, returns to sucking their thumb (flip-flopper) they will have to give the present back to the gift giver until they complete another 10 days and nights in a row with no thumb sucking.

The Second Consecutive 10 Days and Nights
Purpose:
The program continues for a second consecutive 10 days and nights with using only tape on thumb. After successfully completing 20 consecutive days and nights, the parent can gradually reduce the use of tape during the day and or night giving the child more freedom without physical reminders. It takes at least one month to change and stabilize the new pattern. (Read detailed explanation below.)

Procedure:
Continue using the double tape and water-soluble non-toxic markers (same procedure) for the next 10 nights. However, discontinue the elastic bandage (gauze) during the second 10 nights on the program,

After successfully completing the second 10 days and nights the child will receive a second present/reward. If working with a therapist, the child may receive the second present from the therapist. If the parent is initiating the program without professional help, it is recommended the parent provide a second present.

The One Month Rule
In my experience when treating thumb sucking the typically the thumb sucker usually eliminates their thumb sucking within one to three days. However, even if the child stops immediately the program must continue for one full month. **Always One Full Month!**

Purpose
- It takes approximately a month to establish a new pattern.
- It takes a month to stabilize the new pattern.
- Within that month the child will experience an array of feelings: highs and lows, good days and bad, calm and stressful days they

need to navigate without reverting to the coping mechanism of sucking the thumb.
- The child needs to recognize trigger times then utilize coping skills the therapist has introduced.
- When the child spontaneously tells me, "I never think about my thumb anymore," or "I do not have the urge to suck," then I know the child is ready to be dismissed from therapy and have the confidence to maintain this successful non-thumb sucking pattern on their own. The child is ready to graduate.

Program Completion

It is very important to acknowledge successful completion of the thumb program, as well as, express how proud you are of your child's thumb sucking elimination accomplishment. Upon successful completion of this program parents may wish to provide a special gift, a special trophy, if the graduate is a girl a manicure may be a possible choice. As a therapist, I prefer giving the graduate a 'Two Thumb Up' certificate. This certificate not only acknowledges successful thumb elimination, when prominently displayed, represents continuous positive reinforcement.

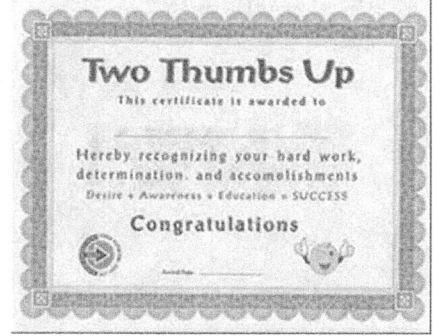

GREAT JOB YOU'VE DONE IT

Parents Executing Thumb Sucking Elimination Program

As a professional who has treated thumb sucking for decades, I have heard a myriad of techniques parents have tried prior to asking for my help. Therefore, I would like to caution parents who are determined to execute this program at home without a therapist's expertise. Experts frequently tell us some children do not fair-well when being helped by parents because they are too close the situation. Sometimes, working with someone outside the family circle has better success. A trained therapist has expertise to evaluate each step, identify triggers causing pitfalls and deal with them. A parent may not recognize these triggers or how to address them.

However, if you are a parent determined to execute a thumb sucking elimination program it is imperative you read the *Two Thumbs*

Up book entirely. It is important parents have empathy and knowledge regarding how and why their child's thumb sucking pattern became chronic. Parents also need to understand what their child is going through physically, emotionally, and chemically before initiating a thumb sucking elimination program This information is detailed in Chapter 6.

In my experience, a thumb sucking elimination program only succeeds, when all facets of the problem are clear, purpose and procedures are understood and executed, and all rules followed by parents and child. The best advice this therapist can provide to parents executing a thumb sucking elimination program; Desire - Awareness - Education = Success. The most important ingredient for success …
'Be Supportive, Be Compassionate and Be Positive.' Always a winning combination.

Chapter 6

The Professional Connection

'Total Patient Care' begins with a Multidisciplinary Approach

Every professional may have their own individual philosophy, regarding as to whether or not a thumb sucking habit needs to be addressed. The chronic thumb sucker may slip through the cracks and is not helped ... or help comes too late with many complications. The purpose of adding 'The Professional Connection' section is to provide detailed information regarding the structural, functional, and chemical changes that occur from chronic sucking patterns and how these changes affect our patients when not addressed.

I would like to introduce the concept of looking at our patients from a perspective of "**Total Patient Care**." Each patient is referred to a specific specialist for a specific issue, however, as health care professionals we need to be aware of '**the total body**' when treating our patients. Ever body part is connected. And one body part will affect other parts of the body compensating by adapting when complications or trauma occur creating a snow ball effect of symptoms and problems that need to be identified through a multidisciplinary approach with the ultimate goal, "**Total Patient Care.**"

Thumb sucking can affect body and mind contributing to physical, emotional, and social complications. If after age three thumb sucking persists, this non-nutritive action may become a habit. This habit may become chronic and detrimental.

Potential Complications from Prolonged Sucking Patterns
- Damage to dentition: Cross bite, excessive over-jet, open bite
- High narrow arched palate
- Nasal cavity may develop a narrow and shallow anatomy
- Low forward rest posture of tongue or tongue thrust
- Abnormal tongue patterns
- Altered respiratory patterns

- Mouth breathing
- Increased freeway space dimension
- Calluses on thumb, finger
- Severe cracked & chapped lips, chapped ring around the mouth
- Skin or cuticle infections
- Difficulty focusing on subject when sucking occurs in school setting
- Reduction of peer acceptance and or bullying
- Germs and illness: do not wash hands before sucking begins
- Speech problems
- Emotional complications affecting patient and siblings

Actual Thumb Sucker Complications

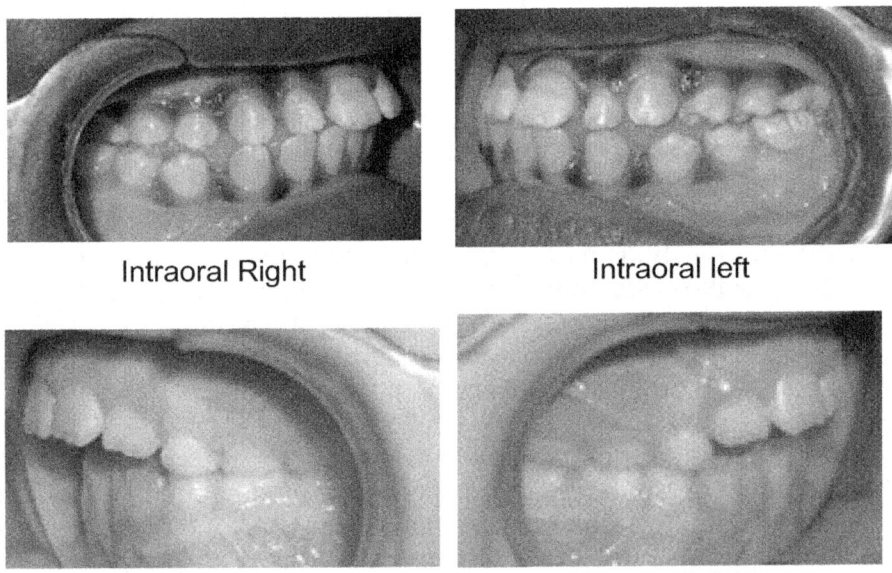

Intraoral Right   Intraoral left

Intraoral left   Intraoral right

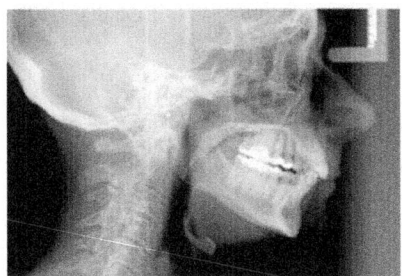 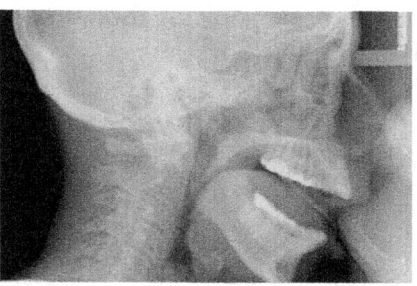

This Cephalogram illustrates a normal rest posture of the lips and normal rest posture of the tongue of a non-thumb sucker

This Cephalogram illustrates a low forward rest posture of the tongue and an increased freeway space when thumb sucking

When you read the long list of potential complications for the patient, the complexity of prolonged sucking patterns become evident: physical, functional, educational, social, emotional, health, and speech.

However, ...*Has anyone ever asked the question, "Can Thumb Sucking Affect the Parent?"*

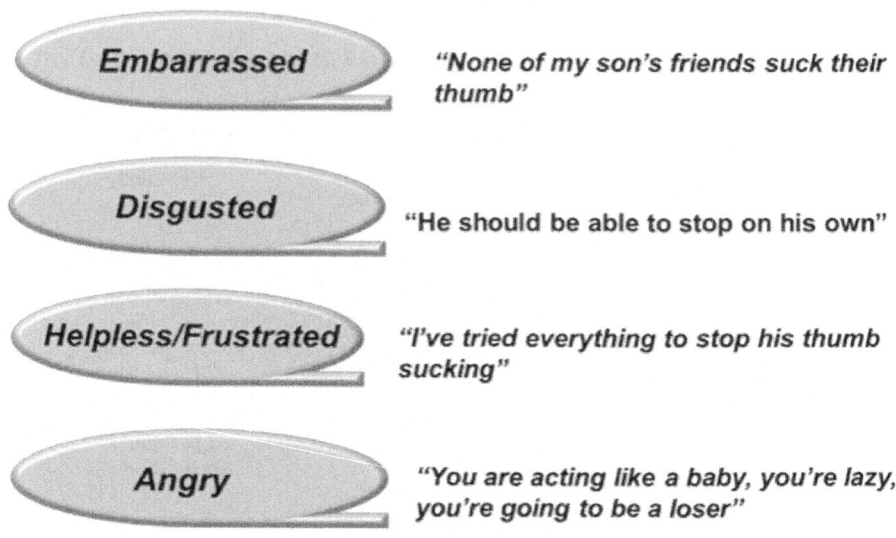

The answer is yes! As professional's we need to recognize all facets of the problem and we need to recognize everyone being affected by

the problem whether directly or indirectly. In other words, we need to take a good look at the *'Whole Picture'* before we set in motion a 'Treatment Plan.'

"It is more than just a simple habit"

Structural - Functional - Chemical Changes

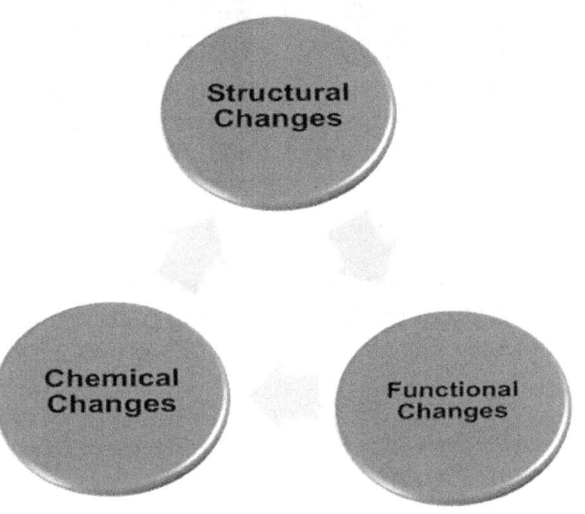

Structural Changes

Forces That Effect Equilibrium and Govern Tooth Position

Intermittent Force	*Governing Forces*	*Continuous Force*
Mastication Swallowing Speaking	Duration of Forces	Orthodontic Appliances
	Pressure From Lips, Cheeks & Tongue	Resting Position Tongue Resting Position Thumb/Finger
Result	External Forces	*Result*
Maintain Equilibrium No Tooth Movement	Eruptive Forces	Alter Previous Equilibrium Tooth Movement

Most Common Damage to the Dentition

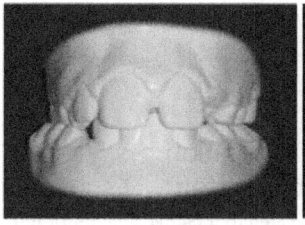
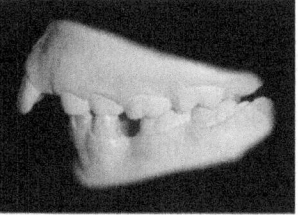

CROSS-BITE   OVERJET

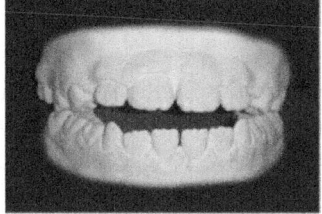

OPEN BITE

Development of other hard structures may become altered in these children.
- The roof of the mouth grows vertically, instead of horizontally; narrows, becomes vaulted, often taking on the shape of the thumb/finger.
- The nasal cavity floor is also associated with growth of the roof of the mouth. If the palate is narrow, the **Nasal Cavity** and **Sinus** may develop a narrow and shallow anatomy.
- With structural changes the tongue moves down and forward opening the dental freeway space (the space between the upper and lower teeth when the mandible is in its physical resting position) beyond its normal dimension. Disruption of normal dental development and over eruption of certain teeth make it possible for abnormal changes in jaw growth to occur.

    Thumb sucking will open the freeway space (opening the mouth) beyond its normal dimension. When the thumb sucking action becomes a set pattern, the tongue adapts to this new low and forward resting position becoming the new normal and will remain low and forward creating an incorrect spring off point triggering changes in chewing, swallowing, speech production and breathing.

The tongue is one of the most adaptable organs in the body. Its main purpose is for survival. If there are airway issues, such as enlarged tonsils and/or adenoids, allergies, or a deviated septum, the tongue will move down and forward opening the freeway space dimension beyond the normal range.

Chemical Changes

We know that tactile stimulation is essential for the development of the central nervous system. Discovering the thumb becomes an extension of mother's feedings, a behavior that becomes automatic. When this non-nutritive action persists, this action becomes a **Habit** and may become chronic and detrimental.

The Central Nervous System produces its own chemical messengers. Pleasurable activities such as running, eating, and thumb sucking stimulate the brain to produce chemical messengers. **Neurotransmitters** are the chemical messengers that are being produced. These neurotransmitter brain chemicals communicate information throughout our brain and body, relaying signals between neurons.

The body uses two types of neurotransmitters which affect the way we act and feel. **Excitatory** increases neurotransmission producing feelings of excitement. Excitatory actions may include sky diving, zip lining, or any activities that produce the sensation of excitement. The second type is **Inhibitory** which decreases neurotransmission producing a calming, relaxed sensation. Inhibitory action may include eating and thumb/finger/tongue sucking actions that produce the sensation of calm, pleasure, comfort and relaxation. Thumb sucking actions also produce **Enkephalins** and **Endorphins** which are the body's natural painkillers.

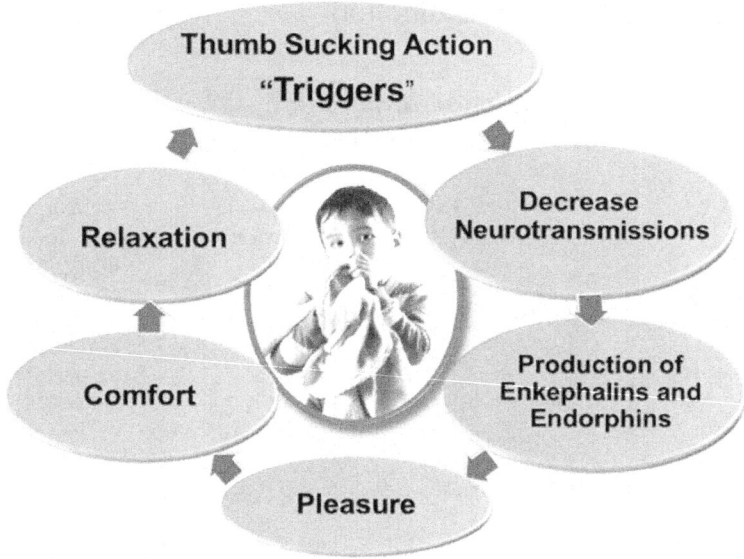

How does this action become a Learned Behavior?

Answer: Operant Conditioning

Learned Behavior

| Pleasure Pain

Reaction

Decreased Neurotransmitter chemicals released | Action Reaction

Reinforces Behavior

Learning Process | Neural pathways form connecting perception reaction

Repetition deepens pathway with similar stimulus | Result

Operant Conditioning

Learned Behavior |

When pleasure or pain is introduced to the brain, the reaction is decreased neurotransmitter chemicals being released. When this occurs, a reaction reinforces the behavior and begins the learning process. Neural pathways form connecting the perception/reaction, then repetition deepens the pathways with repeated similar stimulus. The result is operant conditioning/learned behavior.

How to Achieve Behavior Extinction

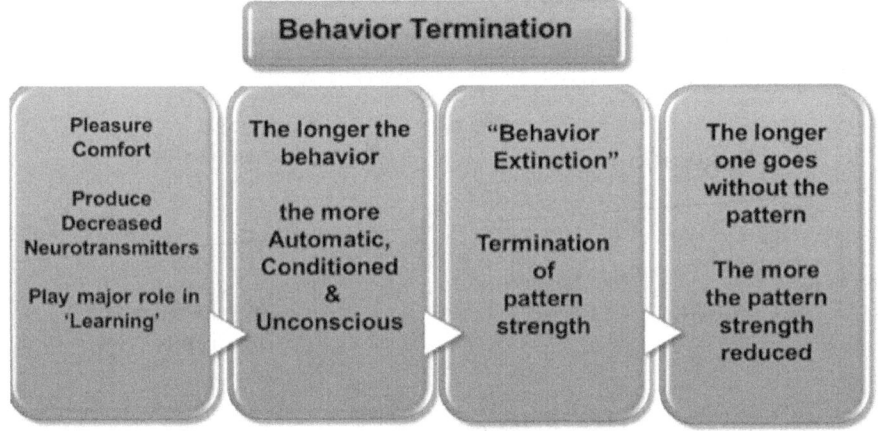

We know pleasure and comfort produce decreased neurotransmitters playing a major role in learning. The longer the behavior continues the more automatic, conditioned and unconscious it becomes.

To achieve behavior extinction, termination of the pattern strength must take place. The longer one goes without the pattern, the more the pattern strength is reduced.

Therapist Role in Behavior Termination
- The brain has '**plasticity**' which means in treatment, skills can be learned to calm the brain's emotional responses and reactive area.
- The therapist has skills to teach the thumb sucker how to enhance their decision-making area instead of responding to the thumb sucking urge impulsively.

Research Pertaining to Decision Making
Neuroscientists at the California Institute of Technology Research have discovered the brain's decision-making spot. Researchers mapped brain activity connecting data with their mapping and connecting performance with certain cognitive tasks. "Caltech researchers could see exactly which parts of the frontal lobe were critical for different tasks like behavioral control." (The research was published in the Proceedings of the National Academy of Sciences.)

Gannon, Megan, "Brain's Decision-Making Spot Found," *Live Science Contributor*, (2012) Aug.21, 03:14pm ET 03:14pm ET
https://www.livescience.com/22570-decisions-controlfrontal- lobe.html

Connecting Cause and Effect

It is important to note what a thumb sucking habit compromises when it becomes a chronic problem. If thumb sucking persists, normal dental equilibrium is disrupted according to Proffit, W.R. & Sarver, H.W., D.M. (207) "Contemporary Orthodontics." *Mosby, Elsevier.*

Stated by Mason, R.M., DMD PhD (2003), "All clinical orthodontics is based on moving teeth by deliberately altering the force applied by the orthodontist to alter the previous equilibrium causing tooth movement" and "The duration of a force, because of the biologic response, is more important that its magnitude." "The timeline for duration to affect the dentition is estimated between four and eight hours." "The perspective offered by Proffit et al., needs to be expanded when considering sucking habits since the negative pressures exerted against the posterior dentition by the cheek muscles during vigorous sucking add an intensity factor not involved in orthodontic treatment. Also, the frequency of the sucking involved whether daytime only, nighttime only, or both, becomes an additional and important consideration."

"If there is a great deal of thumb sucking daily and/or nightly, with a very strong sucking action, and this pattern continues for an extended length of time changes can occur. There can be changes to the dentition and disruption of dental equilibrium (i.e. causing instability of tooth position and interference with the normal rest position of the mandible. The change in the rest posture of the mandible occurs by opening the freeway space which triggers continued eruption of posterior maxillary teeth while the anterior teeth are inhibited from erupting, or the incisors may become flared facially due to the continual presence of a thumb or finger." (Mason, R.M. DMD PhD, 2003)

The constant sucking behavior with the tongue remaining low and forward and the freeway space remaining open for hours per day with a disruption of the dental equilibrium leads to many possible changes involving the orofacial structure, malocclusions, speech problems, and abnormal tongue patterns.

Complications in Speech Production

The facial muscles utilized in chewing, swallowing, and speech constitute an important part of the foundation upon which speech is constructed. When the thumb anchors the tongue down and forward causing an incorrect rest posture of the tongue an inaccurate and inappropriate spring-off point for articulation occurs causing the initiation of the sounds to be misarticulated. Some sounds may be produced incorrectly. When the tongue is resting low and forward, the production of an interdental /t/d/n/l/, and interdental /s/ lisp may occur.

Complications in a School Setting-Social and Emotional

When this chronic behavior occurs in the school environment, children who suck their thumb tend to tune out what is happening around them, lose focus and do not concentrate on school work, and may not participate. It is as if the child is not there; just an empty desk.

All kids want to fit in and have peer acceptance. Being different or doing something not accepted by their peers can lead to being teased, ridiculed, laughed at and, yes, even bullied. How do you think this affects the child's self-esteem?

How many thumb suckers do you know wash their hands before initiating the thumb sucking action? This repetitive sucking behavior exposes them more frequently to germs, dirt, and illness.

Parents and family members may be affected. They become embarrassed, disgusted, angry, and feel helpless and frustrated.

Complications Related to Growth and Development of the Orofacial Structure and Dental Development

If a thumb exerts a force for hours per day against the anterior teeth, positional changes, usually tipping of the teeth, can occur. The most common changes to the dentition include the development of posterior cross-bites, anterior excessive over-jet, and anterior open-bite. The direction of jaw growth may also be negatively affected. The constant pressure of the thumb against the roof of the mouth can also contribute to the development of a narrow, high arched palate. The nasal cavity and sinus can develop a narrow shallow anatomy. Increased freeway space beyond the normal dimension contributes to an open mouth rest posture.

Complications related to Altered Respiratory Patterns

Breathing functions are paramount to health, growth and development and life itself. When normal nasal breathing is disrupted by medical, physical, or environmental factors, compensation and adaptation occurs. The result is habitual mouth-breathing which then continues the snowball momentum leading to multiple problems. Remember, every body part is connected and one body part will affect other parts of the body compensating by adapting when complications or trauma occur creating a snow ball effect of symptoms and problems that need to be identified. Thumb sucking can contribute to airway issues by compromising rest posture of the tongue, lips, body posture, and growth and development of the oro-facial structure.

Today health care professionals are focusing on etiologies, symptoms and complications that occur from persistent constant and habitual mouth-breathing. Pediatric Obstructive Sleep Apnea is being recognized as a crucial problem and needs to be recognized and addressed. When not recognized and addressed, a snowball effect occurs, as already stated, leading to physical and functional changes.

When evaluating a thumb sucking habit other symptoms and complications may be present. These symptoms may or may not be directly related to the reason for the referral. However, as a health care professional we understand multiple complications can develop. Take the time to ask questions (screening) regarding their mouth-breathing and, if concerned, refer to the appropriate professional for evaluation. I am sure you would agree the overall health and well-being of our patients is paramount

Complications Related to Orofacial Myofunctional Disorders (OMD's)

Complications related to OMD's may include postural and functional disorders, inappropriate oral rest postures or functions of the muscles of the tongue, lips, jaw, face, and feeding and swallowing difficulties. Two main causes are thumb sucking and airway issues.

An orofacial myologist is a trained professional who diagnoses and provides treatment for orofacial myofunctional disorders, (OMDs) such as, abnormal tongue patterns, open mouth rest posture of the lips, low forward rest posture of the tongue, and sucking habits. Courses focus on anatomy & physiology, etiologies, signs & symptoms, airway complications all necessary for this professional to provide comprehensive diagnosis and evaluation to treat orofacial myofunctional disorders.

Before an orofacial myologist can begin OMD treatment, sucking patterns (thumb/finger/tongue sucking) habits need to be recognized and addressed. When etiologies, such as sucking patterns, are not addressed, OMD therapy will not be successful. Therefore, as a critical part of orofacial myology education and training all aspects of chronic thumb sucking and successful behavior modification treatment protocols became part of their curriculum. If you would like to learn about orofacial myology the book to read is "Orofacial Myology International Perspectives." (2003) Hanson, M. L., & Mason, R.M., DMD PhD, Thomas, Springfield Illinois.

Does 'All' Thumb Sucking Need to be Addressed?   No.

The following will help you decide if intervention is needed. If the answer to all, some or a few questions is yes, then it is time for action.

Pertinent Questions
- Is there a developing malocclusion – open bite, excessive over-jet, or cross-bite present?
- Does this individual demonstrate a low forward rest posture of the tongue?
- Is there an open mouth rest posture of the lips?
- Are there evident speech problems (i.e., interdental /s/ lisp, /t/, /d/, /n/, and /l/ misarticulation)?
- Is there difficulty in carryover of speech patterns to conversational speech?
- Is there a narrow, high arched palate present?
- Is the thumb sucking strong enough to cause calluses on the sucking digit?
- Is the child's sucking habit resulting in ridicule, harassment, embarrassment or bullying in school?
- Is the child's thumb sucking in school affecting class participation or attention span?
- Has the child expressed interest in eliminating the thumb sucking habit?

How Should It Be Addressed

Now that we know that chronic thumb sucking needs to be addressed and why it needs to be addressed, we need to discuss the **How** it should be addressed.

There are massive amounts of suggestions, advice, recommendations from professionals and laymen, remedies, tools, and gadgets you can browse through on the internet.   After reading awhile your head will spin because you become so confused with choices. Two specific established professional techniques will be discussed along with highlighting positives and negatives of each approach.

Two Professional Techniques
Two well-established thumb elimination techniques are using Habit-Breaking Appliances and Behavior Modification. A detailed description of each technique will be provided followed by comparing the pros and cons of each.

Habit-Breaking Appliance Approach
This approach has been recommended and used for decades by dentists and orthodontists.

Goal of Habit-Breaking Appliance
- Designed to break habits
- Emphasize blocking the thumb or tongue thrust
- Its fixed or removable components can act as mechanical restrainers and muscle retraining devices.

Placement:
"The bands are placed over the maxillary and mandibular anterior teeth. In many cases either just the upper anterior or lower anterior teeth can be used. Prongs or a cage will be attached behind the front teeth. The prongs or cage is to deter the child from putting the thumb in their mouth."

Purpose:
"The purpose of the habit appliance is to help break a thumb habit. The appliance does not prevent placement of the thumb into the mouth, however, it will not feel as comfortable. Prescribed and installed by your health care provider either your dentist or orthodontist." (Technique description came from dental-references.)
https://www.hindawi.com/journals/crid/2013/647649/

Behavior Modification Approach
A behavior modification approach for the treatment of thumb sucking has been recommended and used for decades by professional therapists. Today, with dental specialists recognizing the connection between airway issues and the orofacial complex more and more professionals are embracing the expertise of the Orofacial Myologist. This professional has been trained to address chronic patterns and well versed in behavior modification approaches. A reference book

you may wish to add to your office library *is Fisher, J.E., & O'Donohue, W.T. (2006) "Practioners Guide to Evidence-Based Psychotherapy." College Books Direct.*

Goal of Behavior Modification Approach
To eliminate undesirable habit patterns affecting growth and development that compromise normal functions.

Behavior Modification Approach
Awareness Training:
- It is necessary to know when the thumb sucking occurs. By utilizing behavior modification tools, the longer the child curtails the sucking the more the urge diminishes.
- When using Competing Response Training it is necessary to find something that will effectively curb the undesirable behavior.
- It is imperative to recognize the thumb sucking trigger of the individual child. Finding a replacement behavior, changing the pattern, and having a positive response ready will diminish the child's predisposed behavior of thumb sucking.

Generalization:
- When the habit is eliminated in one situation, you need to make sure it is eliminated in all sucking situations or settings.

To Achieve Habit Reversal
- Motivation enhancement strategies may include wanting to quit for social, behavioral, and or physical reasons.
- Discuss with the child all the pros and cons of NOT sucking their thumb, which might include:
- Social-embarrassment in front of friends, peers or family members
- Social ridicule or rejection inhibit activities and participation (Ex: Uncomfortable attending sleepovers)
- Does not play with friends; too busy sucking thumb
- Physically painful lesions, calluses, infection
- Physical-open bite, over jet, open mouth rest posture of the lips, abnormal tongue patterns, lip incompetence.

Orofacial Myologist
An orofacial myologist is a qualified professional with training to institute a therapeutic program to alleviate a thumb or finger sucking pattern utilizing a **POSITIVE APPROACH**. This professional

evaluates the who, what, when, where, why, before developing and initiating a treatment plan. This treatment includes consultation and evaluation of the child's thumb sucking pattern, addresses the trigger, then maps out an individualized, personalized treatment plan for the thumb sucker.

This behavior modification technique incorporates conscious awareness, motivation and positive reinforcement which includes no negatives, no bad tasting liquid painted on the thumb, no embarrassment, and no punishment. **In most cases the thumb sucking habit can be eliminated within 10 consecutive days and nights.**

Compare Two Professional Techniques

Habit- Breaking Appliance vs. Behavior Modification

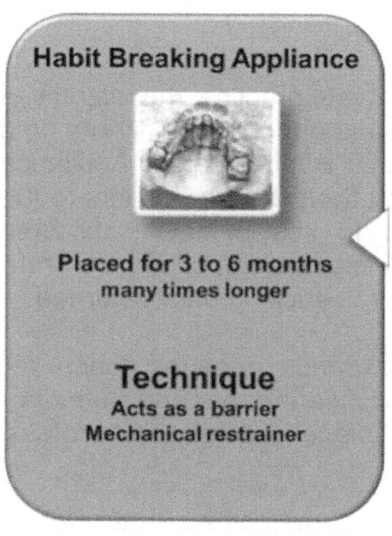

Habit Breaking Appliance

Placed for 3 to 6 months
many times longer

Technique
Acts as a barrier
Mechanical restrainer

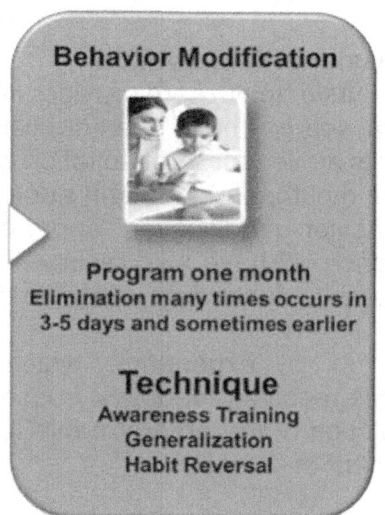

Behavior Modification

Program one month
Elimination many times occurs in
3-5 days and sometimes earlier

Technique
Awareness Training
Generalization
Habit Reversal

Positives and Negatives

Habit Breaking Appliance

Considered a negative by patient

- Appliance blocks the thumb/finger
- Mouth rests open, dropping the tongue
- Compromise speech
- Compromise eating patterns
- Painful

Trigger not addressed
Negative Reinforcement
No compliance needed

Behavior Modification

Considered a positive by patient

- No mechanical devise in mouth
- Mouth rests closed, allowing tongue to rest up
- No speech compromised
- No eating compromised
- No pain

Address the Trigger
Positive Reinforcement
Compliance Needed

Professional Observation

As a health care provider in private practice, the majority of, my referral sources have been dentists and orthodontists. Many potential patients arrived for a consultation with a 'Habit-Breaking Appliance' still in their mouth, and **yes**, **still sucking their thumb.** Others requested a behavior modification approach in lieu of the Habit-Breaking Appliance. I have also received thumb sucking elimination referrals after appliance therapy when the thumb sucking habit returned.

In my experience, which expands decades, once referral sources received feedback from satisfied parents and patients upon completion of the program, this technique became their professional treatment of choice.

I understand many dentists and orthodontists utilize a 'Habit-Breaking Appliance' because it is the treatment protocol most were taught at university and are unaware of any other treatment plan. Every thumb sucker is unique, the reason for sucking is different for each person, and the remedy needs to be individualized as well.

Now that you are aware of an alternative to a Habit-Breaking Appliance and the existence of orofacial myology professionals with special training and expertise in thumb sucking elimination, seek out this professional. Make an appointment, meet, discuss orofacial myology and if you like what you hear, allow this therapist to treat one thumb sucking patient. Upon completion of the program and your patient's positive feedback, I am sure this behavior modification approach will become your treatment of choice.

Chapter 7

Positive Effects of Thumb Sucking

Awareness - Insight - Education

As you know the goal of this book is to provide thumb sucking awareness/insight/education. Experience has taught me nothing is totally positive or negative or totally bad or good. While writing this book, I continued to seek knowledge on all aspects of thumb sucking. I discovered there are positive effects of thumb sucking and fetus research allowed this therapist to expand her awareness and insight of human physiology growth and development. Therefore, this section is dedicated to where it all begins, 'the human fetus.'

Positive Effects of Thumb Sucking

During a class discussion one of my students asked if I had read an article that discussed positive effects of thumb sucking? I said this article was unfamiliar. However, the subject matter peaked my interest. I read the article and wanting to know more, I decided to contact Dr. Carol J. Phillips, who was cited as the original author. After reaching her by phone, a very interesting dialogue ensued. She graciously agreed to be interviewed highlighting the positive effects of thumb sucking. We decided upon a question/answer format.

CSM (Christine Stevens Mills) - "Dr. Phillips, you are a craniosacral therapist, chiropractor, educator, author and owner of 'Dynamic Body Balancing.' Your impressive career has earned you the reputation as an internationally renowned lecturer. Coincidentally, when I mentioned your name to a colleague, I was informed he was a past student of yours. He then continued by saying you were respected by your students and colleagues when he was a student and this respect has expanded to include all health care professionals who have heard you speak.

Question – I would like individuals outside of your professional circle to meet you. In your own words, would you please provide background highlighting your dynamic career?"

Answer - Forty-seven years ago I was a mother with a very sick child. My daughter suffered from a difficult pregnancy, a forceps delivery, a vaccine reaction with her first set of shots, delayed development, intestinal difficulties and chronic ear infections during her first year of life. When she was three, she took a fall from the monkey bars onto her head. This fall resulted in a concussion, vomiting and a loss of reflexes on one side of her body. Nine days later she developed chronic bladder infection that we spent the next three years treating. She eventually lost all bladder control, received a diagnosis of a "neurogenic bladder syndrome" due to severe spasms from the waist down whenever a tablespoon of urine entered her bladder. Eventually, she started to reflux the bacterial infection to her kidneys.

My daughter endured continuous drug therapy and surgical repairs to her urethra to remove the scarring. Fortunately for us, her first-grade teacher strongly recommended chiropractic care to deal with the physical issues and the damaging effects of the drugs she was taking.

Finally, I gave in to my fears and took my daughter to the chiropractor. A simple adjustment to her spine to correct the damaging effects of her delivery and the fall and a recommendation to eliminate all white sugar and white flour led to a speedy and full recovery.

Over the next fifteen years, I completed a degree in Child Development, Chiropractic and Human Service Administration. I then devoted my entire career to practicing and teaching about maternal and child care. A personal experience is the best motivation to become a specialist in a certain area. Don't you agree?"

CSM - "Dr. Phillips, we both agree that every part of the body is connected and dysfunction will affect other parts of the body as we compensate and adapt to trauma."

Question - "What complications or trauma would cause the body to compensate and adapt by triggering a positive thumb sucking response?"

Answer - "To answer this appropriately, we must look to the in-utero experience. If a mother's body is out of balance due to her own birth experience or injuries she has endured prior to or during pregnancy, her uterus will also be out of balance.

If there is any imbalance in the muscles attached to the mother's pelvis (i.e. legs, pelvic floor, spine or abdominal muscles), the uterus, which is anchored securely to the pelvis through a series of strong ligaments, will be distorted. This will result in torsion of the uterine muscles. To accommodate the shape of the mother's distorted uterus, the baby will twist their body to fit within the womb. This compensation pattern alters the baby's ability to maneuver through the birth canal safely and easily. Compensation on the baby's part will also negatively affect the cranial molding process.

During the birth process, cranial molding will allow the cranial plates to overlap and reduce the circumference of the cranium and allow for a smooth transition through the birth canal. Molding of the cranial plates will also reduce the volume of blood and cranial fluid within the cranial vault by pushing it down into the spinal canal. If the baby is in the proper position for birth, uterine contractions will slowly and precisely force the head and neck into flexion, stack up the cervical vertebra, open the foramen and prevent any pressure on the cranial nerves. Anything other than this normal flexion of the body with the head tucked tightly into the chest and extremities folded tightly into their chest, will result in abnormal molding and a subsequent restriction in the flow of vascular and Cerebral Spinal Fluid."

Question - "How does thumb sucking help restore balance to the craniosacral system?"

Answer - "After birth, the baby will take their first breath and begin the process of unfolding the cranial plates, which are floating on the dura. This unfolding process will restore balance to the flow of cranial fluids within the brain and around the spinal cord. If distortion occurred due to restriction within the baby's musculoskeletal system, the flow of blood and cranial fluid will be diminished. Sucking immediately helps restore balance within the dural membranes. If the cranial plates are overlapped and locked into an aberrant position, the baby will want to suck constantly, even though there is no milk production. As they mature and have better control of their nervous system, they will often need a pacifier to be soothed. If there is extreme distortion around the Hypoglossal Nerve, the tongue will not be able to pull the pacifier into their mouth and the baby will cry and appear to reject it. Eventually, the baby will get the motor control needed to suck their own thumb or fingers to put the cranial base into motion.

Thumb sucking will result in a lifting of the maxilla and vomer at the roof of the mouth. The vomer will then apply pressure to the sphenoid and set the sphenoid and occiput into motion. This movement of the cranial base will bathe the brain and spinal cord with cerebral spinal fluid (nutrients) and restore adequate reabsorption of waste products back into the vascular system. If the sphenoid and occiput don't move freely, none of the cranial, spinal or pelvic bones move adequately. Thumb sucking is a survival technique and will continue into adulthood if the musculoskeletal restriction is not reduced or eliminated. We must use obsessive nursing, pacifier use and chronic thumb sucking as an indicator for cranial and spinal restrictions that are reducing the flow of CSF and blood around the brain and spinal cord."

CSM - "I want to thank Dr. Phillips for participating in this question/answer dialogue providing the reader insight to positive effects of thumb sucking."

As health care professionals, we need to listen to each patient then consistently consider the premise of cause and effect. Background and symptoms provide the clues. As professionals we need to recognize those clues. A child with a chronic thumb sucking pattern, a high narrow palate, open mouth rest posture, a low forward rest posture of the tongue, and or possible speech problems will need a multi-disciplinary approach to evaluate all contributing factors. A multi-disciplinary approach provides additional insight to expand upon and interpret before mapping out a treatment approach. Further research can lead to discovery and expansion of knowledge, establish or confirm facts, all of which can lead to solving new or existing problems.

The Need to Suck

What has past research taught us? Sucking is a reflex, it is normal and natural and a necessity for survival. Sucking provides tactile stimulation essential for development of the central nervous system. Infants have a built-in need and enjoy sucking. Newborns come equipped with two specific innate reflexes, rooting and sucking. Both are necessary for survival. Rooting prepares the baby to suck and sucking begins when the roof of the mouth is touched stimulating the automatic response to suck. Sucking becomes coordinated with swallowing and breathing. The development of or lack of development provides information telling us if the central nervous system is developing normally.

Research: Durham University

Research regarding fetuses/babies continues to add to our understanding of pre and post birth development and physiology. The more we know what is 'normal', the more we can predict, prepare and address what is 'abnormal.'

Research at Duke University, led by Dr. Nadja Reissland from the Department of Psychology, has been researching 'fetus' physiology. Dr. Reissland states, "By building upon previous research, we prepare the child for life outside the womb." (8 October 2013, Babies learn to anticipate touch in the womb.) Recent research by her team observed, "Increased touching of the lower part of the face and mouth in fetuses could be an indicator of brain development necessary for healthy development, including preparedness for social interaction, self-soothing and feeding."

Dr. Reissland and her research team at Durham state, "The latest findings could improve understanding about babies, especially those born prematurely, their readiness to interact socially and their ability to calm themselves by sucking on their thumb or fingers." Research showed that Gestation by 36 weeks, fetuses were opening their mouths prior to the mouth being touched which the team interpreted, at this stage, had "awareness of mouth movements." "Previous theories suggested that 'movement in sequence' could form the basis for the development of intention in fetuses."

"Early on in development, babies were more likely to touch the upper and side parts of the face, however, when older their thumbs reliably targeted the mouth." "Between 24-36 weeks there seemed to be a transition from hitting the top of the head to the mouth." Dr Nadja Reissland continued by stating, "Observing when fetuses open their mouths before sucking their thumbs could be a test of development." LENNART NILSSON/REUTERS October 9 2013, The Times).

"As baby learns a great deal through the tactile sensations in his mouth (which is why your newborn and young baby will often be seen exploring by putting things into their mouth) this gradually leads to learning how to suck their thumb." Reissland, N. (2013).

During ultrasounds the images of fetuses have been viewed sucking their thumb. This illustrates during the fetal stage of development the thumb is discovered and thumb sucking can begin pre-birth. We also know that thumb sucking triggers the comfort feeling and relieves pain and stress.

Janet DiPietro a Johns Hopkins University psychologist along with other researchers, state "At 32 weeks of gestation--two months before a baby is considered fully prepared for the world, or "at term" --a fetus is behaving almost exactly as a newborn. And it continues to do so for the next 12 weeks."
https://www.psychologytoday.com/us/articles/199809/fetal-psychology

Research continues to provide more information about growth and development and similarities of this sucking action pre and post birth. This makes one pause and wonder, if this action begins pre-birth and continues post-birth could thumb sucking be "More than just a simple habit?"

Research References:
https://www.dur.ac.uk › Durham University News ›

https://www.dur.ac.uk/news/newsitem/?itemno=18810

https://medicalxpress.xncom%20%20psychology%20%26%20psychiatr-m75w/

https://www.google.com/search?q=LENNART+NILSSON%2FREUTERS+October+9+2013%2C+The+Time&oq=LENNART+NILSSON%2FREUTERS+October+9

http://voxhumanaenglish.com/Newest%20Science%20News%20Blog%2020131014.pdf

https://www.dur.ac.uk/news/newsitem/?itemno=18810%20

https://medicalxpress.com/news/2013-10-babies-womb.html This research published in the journal "Developmental Psychobiology."

Chapter 8

Laughter Makes us Healthier

As professionals, taking care of patients is very important. However, equally important is **You, The Professional.** Therefore, this next section is dedicated to your health and well-being. A sense of humor, a smile and a laugh, will help to create a positive attitude. A positive attitude can impact every aspect of your life.

Laughter - Physical Health Benefits
- Laughter boosts the immune system by decreasing stress hormones and increases immune cells and infection-fighting antibodies improving your resistance to disease.
- Laughter lowers stress hormones by relaxing the whole body, relieves physical tension and stress, and leaves your muscles relaxed for up to 45 minutes after.
- Laughter decreases pain by triggering the release of endorphins promoting an overall sense of well-being and can even temporarily relieve pain.
- Laughter protects the heart by improving the function of blood vessels and increases blood flow, which can help protect against a heart attack and other cardiovascular problems.
https://www.mayoclinic.org/healthy-lifestyle/stress- management

Laughter - Mental Health Benefits
- Laughter eases anxiety and tension by stopping distressing emotions. It is very difficult to feel anxious, sad or angry when laughing.
- Laughter helps us relax by reducing stress and increasing energy enabling us to stay focused and accomplish more.
- Laughter helps us maintain or improve our perspective by allowing us to see things from a realistic perspective instead of feeling overwhelmed.
https://www.helpguide.org/articles/mental-health/laughter-is-the-best-medicine.htm

Laughter is and always will be the best form of therapy

For four decades I have enjoyed working with children who suck their thumb. One of my favorite parts of the consultation is asking the following questions. "Why do you suck your thumb?" "What have you done to try to stop?" And my all-time favorite, "What does your thumb taste like?

Here is what some of my clients have said:

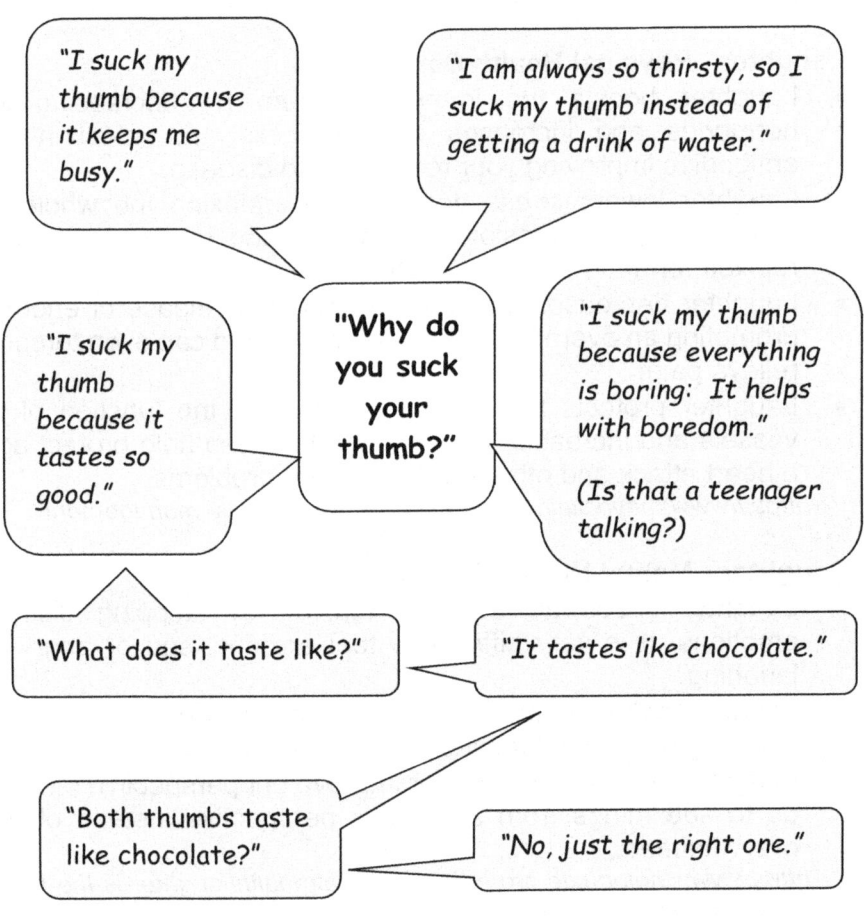

**The remedies others have admitted to are even better…
From parents:**

"I have tried dunking my child's thumb in hot sauce."

My response - **"All this does is give your child an acquired taste for Mexican Food."**

Others have tried placing a sock over the whole hand.

My response - **"This makes for a soggy sock," "Must be a new twist on "Open mouth and insert foot."**

One of the most unusual remedies I have heard was that of putting a boxing glove on both hands to prevent the thumb from entering the mouth.

My response - "**Be careful, I warned. Your child just might knock himself out. I guess that is one way to solve the problem!"**

Chapter 9
Case Studies

Reading a book about thumb sucking elimination which addresses the physical, emotional, and social ramifications, the chemical components, the step-by-step procedures, the recommendations and cautions are all just words until you personalize it. The case studies that follow illustrate **Awareness + Education + Cooperation + Compassion** result in the perfect formula for thumb sucking elimination success, but because each person involved has their own story behind their subsequent thumb sucking, the approaches and rate of achievement will differ. *Names have been changed, as well as, selective history & background omitted for confidentiality.*

Case Study 1
Girl age 5
Thumb Sucker with Severe Open Bite
Background:
It was a typical morning at my office. I always arrived an hour early to check messages and do paper work. I had not been working more than fifteen minutes when the phone rang. It was a local dentist, Dr. Richards. I recognized his name immediately. Within the dental field he is a well-known and respected dentist with a very large preventive dentistry practice. Dr. Richards works with young children to alleviate problems that contributed to preventing natural growth and development. He asked to make an appointment for his five-year-old daughter who sucks her thumb.

He said, "I am very concerned about my daughter's severe open bite at such an early age. She sucks her thumb all day long, when trying to go to sleep, and the entire time she is asleep. She loves her thumb."

I explain, "In many cases when thumb sucking is stopped at an early age, natural growth and development can continue allowing the open bite to either close down or at least improve. Prolonged thumb or digit sucking can contribute to not only dental problems, compromise growth and development of the orofacial structure, compromise speech production, change functional nasal breathing into mouth breathing, contributing to changes in rest posture of the tongue, and the list goes on." After discussing the complexities of prolonged thumb sucking Dr. Richards made an appointment for his daughter Katie.

Consultation:

Katie and Dr. Richards arrive on time for their 3:30 p.m. appointment. I like to observe my prospective clients in my waiting room before I begin a consultation. It is a standard routine in my practice. A great deal of insight can be learned through observation. I immediately notice that Dr. Richards appears to be a very loving father for he is laughing and joking with Katie. I notice this puts her at ease. Katie appears to be a very vivacious, wide-eyed blond, attentive, listening to her father and sucking her thumb intensely. I greet the Richards and invite them to follow me into my office. When they entered the office, Dr. Richards asks Katie to take her thumb out of her mouth. She smiles and does as he asks.

I proceed to ask Katie some questions to help her relax. "How was school?"

She said, "It was a fun day."

I then ask Katie if she knows why she is here? I like to ask, for if the individual will not admit there is a sucking problem, we will not be able to begin a program. I speak directly to Katie. If Katie answers most questions instead of waiting for dad to do the talking, she is probably mature enough for the thumb sucking elimination program. How she answers the questions also informs me how motivated she is to want to try to stop. It is important to get an understanding of how the patient feels, not how Mom or Dad feel.

I want Katie to understand the consequences of prolonged thumb sucking. I illustrate the consequences through show and tell. I place different models of malocclusions and one beautiful set of teeth on my desk and ask, "Which set of teeth would you like to have when you are an adult?" In Katie's case she points to the beautiful set of teeth and we then discuss what needs to happen for her to have teeth like that.

I like to ask a series of questions. (Questions to determine the child's readiness are listed in Chapter 2) I like to add humor to my questions. I ask younger clients, "What does your thumb taste like?" In Katie's case I think you will chuckle over her answer.

Question: "Katie, do you like to suck your thumb?"
Answer: "Yes!"

Question: "What does your thumb taste like?"
Answer: "It tastes like chocolate."

Question: "Both thumbs taste like chocolate?"
Answer: "No, just the right one!"

Katie tells me that she would like to stop sucking her thumb and that she likes coming to my office. She is a sweet little girl motivated to stop sucking her thumb and said she would like my help. That is the first step to success.

Results:
I never begin a program at the initial consultation. I use the initial visit to get to know the potential patient and the patient to feel comfortable with me. I also ask if she likes to hold something when she sucks her thumb, which is known as a 'trigger.' Katie's preference was a stuffed hippo name Geraldine. I ask Katie to bring Geraldine to her next appointment. Katie said she would be glad to bring Geraldine to meet me.

On the second visit, Katie arrives with Geraldine and both parents. I ask Katie if she is ready to give up her thumb sucking, and she strongly says, "YES."

I then have a chat with her friend Geraldine. I tell Geraldine, "You are very cute, I know you are a very good friend to Katie." I then ask Geraldine if she has ever gone on vacation without Katie?
Katie jumps in and tells me, "Geraldine has only been on vacation with us."
I then ask Katie, "Don't you think Geraldine is old enough to have her own vacation?" I explain that it would make it easier for Katie to stop thumb sucking if Geraldine went on vacation while we were in a thumb sucking elimination program. I know Geraldine is a friend, but she is also a 'trigger.' I explain when Geraldine is being held by Katie the urge to suck her thumb is very strong. I suggest, "Let's allow

Geraldine to go on a wonderful vacation and Katie can choose Geraldine's vacation destination." Katie understands that we are not getting rid of Geraldine (which would be a negative), but we are rewarding Geraldine by allowing her to have an adventure (which is a positive) while Katie has her own adventure of thumb sucking elimination.

Katie agrees, Geraldine goes on vacation and Katie's program begins. Katie is asked to make a Spoon Person and a thumb chart and bring them to our next appointment. Spoon Person and Thumb Chart are explained in Chapter 5) I also tell the family that if Katie wants to call to tell me she is doing great, please let her. I then set up the next appointment and ask if there are any unanswered questions? I give Katie a hug before the family leaves.

Katie arrives to her next appointment carrying her thumb chart, her Spoon Person, tape and marker on her thumb and a big smile on that beautiful face. Katie is beaming. She tells me she did not suck her thumb since I saw her last.

"Geraldine is having fun at the beach on her vacation and I named my spoon person Star."

"I ask her why she named her Star?"

Katie replies, "I named her Star because she helped me get seven stars on my chart."
I ask Katie, "How do you feel now that you have not sucked your thumb for seven days and nights?"

She says, "It was easier than I thought, and I am having fun!"
I ask Dr. & Mrs. Richards how they feel Katie is doing? "She is sleeping well, happy to go to bed, and her attitude during the day has been great," they reply.

Katie completed her thumb program successfully within one month. She was a pleasure to work with. Dad was so pleased with the positive approach and successful outcome he continues to refer patients to me regularly.

Case Study 2
Girl age 15
Pacifier Sucking Problem with Severe Open Bite
Background:

I thought I had heard everything until an orthodontist called and proceeded to tell me he has a young patient with a severe open bite and still sucks on a pacifier.

He explained to the family before he can begin orthodontics she has to give up the pacifier. Tiffany irritated, emphatically denied pacifier sucking and sounded very defensive. Mrs. Russell interrupted her daughter and proceeded to tell me that Tiffany not only sucks the pacifier, she throws a tantrum when a family member tries to take the pacifier away from her.

Dr. Owens was sympathetic yet firm explaining Tiffany had to stop before getting braces. He told them he could not help her with the pacifier problem however, he knew someone who might be able to help. He would discuss her case, with their permission, then get back with them.

I said, "I would be happy to consult but would not decide, as to whether I would take Tiffany on as a client or to refer her to another professional until we met and had a consultation.

When meeting Tiffany she appeared to be a very outgoing teenager. I asked her what activities she was interested in?

"She said I am very active at school, on the debate team, volleyball team and a cheerleader."

After some generic questions, I asked Tiffany, "Why did you come to see me?"
Her response was, "She didn't know."

I already knew that was untrue after discussing the case with Dr. Owens. I move on even though she does not acknowledge she sucks on a pacifier. I will come back to this point again later when she feels more comfortable with me. I explain about my therapy program and answer questions. Then I explain I do not want to begin a program today but would like to see Tiffany next week allowing her time to think about our discussion and decide if she would like my help.

Upon the second visit Tiffany was open and comfortable, however, she continued to say she did not know why she was at my office. We talked for approximately a half hour and before we ended our visit I expressed to Tiffany that I was there to help her if she wanted my help, but she had to tell me why she was at my office first. I also explained to Mrs. Russell and Tiffany that I would be willing to set up one more appointment. However, if Tiffany did not acknowledge she needed my help and for what, I would not begin a program and would recommend they seek help elsewhere, possibly a psychiatrist or psychologist.

Upon the third visit, I ask Mrs. Russell and Tiffany to decide if they want to meet with me together, or if Tiffany would like to meet with me by herself (with mom's permission). Both feel it would be beneficial if I talk to Tiffany alone.

By this time Tiffany was comfortable with me. She proceeds to tell me how her volleyball team is doing and what she did over the weekend. She then tells me she wants my help to stop sucking her pacifier. I told her that is half the battle, to admit there is a problem and acknowledge she wants to stop. We can now begin to work together.

I explain she needs to give up the pacifier cold turkey. I suggest we have a good-bye ritual then retire the pacifier. I also ask Tiffany to make a chart to plot each successful day she completes without the pacifier. If Tiffany is willing to follow my directions to the letter and we work together, as a team, she will achieve her goal of giving up the pacifier.

I discuss a reward system with Mrs. Russell and Tiffany. In my experience rewarding determination and hard work provides a formula for success.

I suggest Tiffany check in with me at the end of each day to give me an update on her progress. Checking in helps to keep the individual motivated.

Tiffany says, "I will be her crisis line and she likes the idea that she can reach me any time, if needed, as well as tell me how well she does each day."

I see Tiffany a week later and she is beaming with delight. She called me every day that week to tell me how well she was doing. However, when we have our visit she goes into extensive detail regarding the exit of the pacifier. She went all out. "I took a small box, made a paper heart and glued it to the lid of the box. I then placed the pacifier in it and secured the box with tape. Mom and I had a little ritual in my room where I said good-bye to the pacifier and placed it in the garbage for pick up the next morning."

On our last visit Tiffany completed a month with no pacifier. Mom said, "Tiffany is happy and continues to be very active."

Tiffany said, "I now feel like a grown up and proud of what I have accomplished." "I do not think about the pacifier anymore."

Before mom left my office, she wanted to speak with me alone. She said, "We are extremely happy with how well the program worked." "No more pacifier-no more tantrums." This pattern ceased the day she threw the pacifier away.

Case Study 3
25-year-old male
Thumb Sucker with Excessive Overjet

Background:
Most people are very surprised by my answer to this question, "How old is the oldest individual that has come to you for help to stop a thumb or digit pattern? When I say the oldest thumb sucking person I have ever treated was fifty-six years old I immediately see eyes widen and jaw drops.

I received a phone call from a 25-year-old male who was referred to my clinic by his orthodontist. Mr. Dan explained he went to an orthodontist because he wanted a better smile.

During the consultation with the orthodontist Dan was asked point blank, "Do you suck your thumb?"

"Boy was I surprised at that question." No one in years had asked me if I still suck my thumb including my parents." I then told Dr. Banks the orthodontist, "Yes I do." I continued by asking him, "How did you know I still suck my thumb?" He proceeded to explain that due to his excessive overjet and cross-bite it was obvious. Dr. Banks explained that he could not begin any orthodontic treatment until the thumb sucking stopped.

Dan was very open regarding the purpose of his consultation with me and that is always a good sign. I told Mr. Dan to relax and tell me in his own words his concerns.

Dan's dialogue… I listened while he provided his thumb sucking history. "I sucked on a pacifier until age 5. At age 5 the pacifier was taken away by my parents. I immediately started sucking my thumb. I sucked during the day, at school and to get to sleep. I was badly teased at school for sucking my thumb. I could see this memory was very troubling for him to talk about. Kids at school teased me on the playground, calling me a baby. I would become so upset I would get into fights with the guys that teased me. That was unacceptable behavior with the school and my parents. After being punished for getting into fights I was determined to, at least, stop sucking my thumb at school. However, I continued to suck in the privacy of my home after school and at bed time. During my teenage years it got even worse. I would hide it from my parents. It was very difficult for me because I felt isolated from my friends, different, alone, and embarrassed. "Being a teenager is difficult enough without adding peer pressure to the mix. As an adult, I was too embarrassed to ask for help, let alone know who or where to get that help."

"After the orthodontic consultation, I understood the necessity of alleviating the thumb pattern before braces could be put on. It is obvious to me that my thumb sucking habit which developed at an early age has caused many complications and I am ready to get rid of that habit."

I explain to Dan that he is not alone. I have helped many adults eliminate their thumb sucking. My practice specializes in the treatment of orofacial myofunctional disorders. My training included education and treatment of thumb/finger and tongue sucking. I mention the oldest adult I have helped, so far, has been fifty-six years old. Dan looked surprised. I wanted Dan to feel comfortable and understand that he is not the only adult that sucks his thumb, so there is no reason to be embarrassed.

I expressed that asking for help to stop thumb sucking is the first step. "You have the right attitude and seem very determined." You are ready and willing to stop this habit. Let's begin.

Results:
Dan began his program the following week. He stopped thumb sucking within 10 days and was very pleased with his progress and looked forward to beginning orthodontic treatment. I continued to see him once a week for a month until he felt confident he could successfully maintain on his own.

Post therapy:
I received a very nice phone call from Dan a few years later. He said he wanted to thank me for my help. He was out of braces and wearing a retainer. His teeth looked great; he got a new job and was now engaged. All in all, a very happy young man with what sounds like a very bright future.

Case study 4
Boy age 6
Right/ Left Thumb/Finger Sucker with Open bite

A previous client's mother, Mrs. Holiday called and asked if I would be willing to see one of her neighbors. She told her neighbor Carolyn about her son's visits with me and how I helped him stop his thumb sucking pattern in ten days. The neighbor immediately wanted my number for she had been trying to get Tim to stop his thumb sucking forever.

When Tim and Mrs. Street arrived I immediately took a liking to him. Tim is a very happy go lucky, energetic, friendly little boy. However, when he smiled I could see a severe open bite. I could tell Tim was comfortable in his surroundings, it appeared he would be comfortable anywhere he was. He is just that type of kid.

When Tim sat down, I noticed he had his hands up on his face, then on his head, then he pulled his ears before putting his hands back on his face. I knew this was going to be a problem. I thought I would ask Mrs. Street for some background while I continued to observe Tim.

Background:
Mrs. Street proceeded to tell me, "Tim prefers to suck his left thumb however, he will switch from the left thumb to the right thumb. If neither are available, he will then move on to whatever finger was available on either hand. Sucking since birth, he has two favorite blankets, as well as, soft stuffed animals he likes to hold when

sucking. His sucking occurs during the day-at school-when going to bed-and while asleep."

Consultation:
While mom is talking I continued watching Tim, who slowly moves his hands to eye level then, before you know it, his hands are on his face and the right thumb sneaks into his mouth. The target destination is achieved. Mom asks him to remove the thumb and in a couple of minutes, he repeats this action. I see a pattern emerging. Mom says she is concerned because his teeth are moving.

I see pros and cons to beginning a program with this child. The pros are as follows: He is a very outgoing, pleasant, happy little boy. He acknowledged he wants to stop sucking his thumb and understands he is messing up his teeth. The cons to beginning the program are as follows: I observe Tim cannot keep his hands away from his face. This could be a real obstacle to a successful program, due to the fact, when hands are constantly near the mouth the thumb or fingers can sneak in without being noticed.

I explain the program to Tim and his mom emphasizing how important following the rules are and for Tim to have success in this program we need to work together finding ways to keep his hands away from his face. Tim agrees, and we decide to begin the thumb program on his next visit. I think what impressed me the most and swayed my decision to begin was the fact Tim was so enthusiastic about wanting to stop and willing to cooperate. The desire, awareness and education lay the ground work for a successful program.

Results:
Tim has not sucked his thumb-fingers at school; he has not sucked his thumb-fingers falling asleep or while asleep. However, he has slipped twice at home during the day within the first seven days on the program. We talked about the slips and why it may have happened. I then give him suggestions to help him during the day and a pep talk explaining we all slip sometimes. I tell him, if he gets the urge to suck or just wants to tell me how well he is doing, call me. "I am always here for you". "Stay positive".

Tim is trying very hard, is cooperative, and considering the severity of this thumb-finger pattern he has done extremely well in a short period of time. His parents and I have praised him for his partial success and have expressed he has conquered half of the problem (keeping it positive). We now will work on the other half. Keeping his hands away from his face is his biggest obstacle.

After two months of not sucking, no fingers, no thumbs, nothing at all Tim was very pleased with himself and both parents were thrilled.

Tim then told me, "I don't think about my thumb or fingers anymore." Mom told me she never sees him with his hands anywhere near his face. This was an important positive change in his behavior.

Remember, no two thumb or finger suckers are alike. You need to treat every single case as special. Not every case will have immediate success. When a slip occurs, it is the job of the trained therapist to look at the pattern, ask pertinent questions, formulate a plan, make adjustments when necessary, then help the patient execute the plan.

Keeping the patient and family positive is a key factor. I have learned, when one does not achieve success immediately, or encounter pitfalls along the way disappointment sneaks in and needs to be addressed before the decision to give up occurs. It's the therapist's job to be the cheerleader helping to keep everyone optimistic and moving forward to achieve the goal. After forty years of treating thumb and finger sucking there are still cases that challenge me. "That is what keeps life interesting don't you think"?

Case Study 5
Boy age 7
Traveler to Mom & Dad's Bed Thumb Sucker with Open Bite

When every therapist begins his/her career we fear there will be that one unique case, that unusual case that become a true challenge. And that is what occurred when little Trenton was referred to me.

Background:
Trenton is a sweet, happy go lucky little boy that sucks his right thumb, day, night, when bored, tired, watching T.V., going to sleep and while asleep.

Consultation:
During the consultation I asked Trenton about his thumb sucking. "I suck my thumb when trying to go to sleep and while

asleep." Then mom interjected some additional facts that Trenton left out of the story.

Mom told me, "Trenton does not stay in his own bed at night. He starts out sleeping in his own bed, but then wakes up, walks down the hall to our bedroom, then gets into bed with us and puts his thumb back in his mouth to fall back to sleep."

I then ask, "How often does Trenton come to your bed?"

The answer is, "Almost every night!" But that is, 'not all of the story'. Trenton not only comes to our bed, he wakes his little brother and has him accompany Trenton to our bed.

No, that is not the end of the story. Mom is now pregnant with their third child. Their bed is 'definitely' crowded and something needs to change before the new baby arrives. Not only for Trenton but for the well- being of the whole family.

Treatment Plan:
Mom and dad are willing to do whatever asked of them during the thumb program and Trenton is very eager to stop. Mom asks, "Can we begin a thumb treatment program with Trenton right now"?

"I answer, **No.** First, Trenton has to learn to stay in his own bed all night."

"Why does he first have to stay in his own bed before beginning the thumb program?"

My reasoning:
When a nighttime thumb therapy program begins the patient needs to start and stay in their own bed (all night). When Trenton wakes up, he gets out of his bed and goes to mom and dad's bed. Once he reaches his destination, climbs in their bed, the thumb returns to his mouth, reverting to the familiar set pattern of sucking to relax, allowing him to fall asleep again.

For a program to be successful all '**triggers**' need to be addressed and a regular routine and rules need to be followed. Going to Mom and Dad's bed is a trigger for Trenton and to fall back to sleep he will put his thumb in to relax. (The trigger and all rules are discussed in the book.)

Before we begin the thumb program I set up a one week **'no mom & dad's bed'** reward program. Trenton makes a chart where he can track his progress. He places a star on his chart each morning for staying in his own bed. I make a deal with Trenton that if he completes seven successful nights he will receive a prize from me (as a reward.) He agrees and says he will call me each morning to tell me he got a whole star on his chart.

After a week of straight stars, we are ready and able to begin Trenton's thumb elimination program. Trenton did equally well with the thumb program.

Mom and Dad are very proud of Trenton and extremely grateful Trenton and his brother are no longer occupying their bed. I told Trenton he grew up before my eyes, sleeping in his own bed and no more thumb sucking. I am very, very, proud of him.

I then tell him, "You will be a great big brother when the new baby arrives".

Case Study 6
Girl age 10
Habit-Breaking Appliance Thumb Sucker- Switch Hitter

Background:
- Sucking thumb in womb. Father brought in ultrasound of sucking child
- Will switch from sucking right thumb to the left thumb
- Sucks day, night, used to suck at school but stopped this year
- Triggers: Plays with belly button while sucking her thumb
- Referred by orthodontist

Methods tried to help Olivia stop:

I ask dad, "What remedies have you tried to help Olivia stop her thumb sucking?"

Dad replies, "Everything! Gloves on hands, long talks, flavoring on thumb, rewards, punishment, thumb guards, and then a Habit-Breaking Appliance was placed in her mouth. It worked for a couple of days then she learned how to work around it and went back to sucking with the appliance."

Comments after Thumb Elimination Therapy:

Dad speaking:
"I felt the program was very worthwhile. After exhausting all other attempts at trying to help Olivia stop sucking her thumb it was a relief that something finally worked.
"I would highly recommend this program. After 10 years of sucking her thumbs we came to you, began a program, it was easy, fun, and successful. We are very grateful! We are all very happy with her success."

Case Study 7
Presented in Letter Form
Mom's letter "Parents want choices"
A Habit Breaking Appliance case

"Tom is my son who is now 11 years old. When he was born he weighed 8 lbs.,6 oz's. So, he wasn't really that little. Once Tom started to walk and run around, he trimmed down. According to the growth and weight charts that were done every year by his pediatrician (at his well visits), Tom was following a steady curve of weight but, a little slower growth, although still only being in the 25th percentile."

"By the time he was nine years old, like most, he needed braces. We went to see an orthodontist. Before he could have braces put on, he needed an expander. Not only an expander, but a habit breaking appliance with it. The appliance will be put on when the expander goes on, 'To break an unwanted habit.'

Tom had his expander and habit appliance installed. The assistant at the orthodontist office explained, "That it will take some time getting used to this appliance, but shouldn't take too long."

I understood what they said, yet, "I still couldn't help feeling, that this was some kind of cruel punishment. I wish there were some other way of going about this."

"Tom seemed to deal with it, probably better than I at first, until it came to his eating. We cut food up into very small bites so that he would have an easier time chewing and swallowing. Even spaghetti, cut up gave him problems. He felt like he was gagging on it. After that, he wouldn't eat spaghetti at all.

Eating got easier, because now Tom was choosier on what he would eat. There were foods that he refused to eat, no matter how small we cut it, he was afraid of it getting caught on the appliance and making him gag."

Tom went back to his pediatrician, this time there was a change in Tom's weight chart. He fell off the graph! He had lost weight and the only thing that was different from the last visit, was the habit appliance.

Upon Tom's next orthodontic appointment, "I asked if there was something else that could be used instead of the habit appliance? I wanted it off."

That is when he was referred to Chris an orofacial myologist for treatment.

"We would have to travel about 40 miles to the appointment, but I said it will be well worth the miles. Anything so Tom wouldn't have to wear that appliance. We were grateful to know there was an alternative to the appliance and the alternative did not hurt and worked."
Signed, Mom

Note:
"This is an unusual case, however, wouldn't it have been nice if the parents and patient were provided treatment options earlier rather than later?"

Two Thumbs Up A - Guide for Parents/Patients/Professionals

Two Thumbs Up is an accumulation of Christine's experiences and orofacial myology expertise comprised of forty years in private practice, eighteen years teaching at University of Detroit Mercy orthodontic department, and teaching COM® (Certified Orofacial Myologist) Certification Track Courses.

Two Thumbs Up understanding and treatment of thumb sucking a Guide for Parents and Professionals by Christine Stevens Mills takes an in-depth look at the complexity of thumb sucking, complications and ramifications related to the oro-facial structures and beyond. Connections are made between chronic sucking patterns and possible changes in structures and functions, breathing patterns, rest postures, speech, and unrealized educational, social, emotional, and family dynamic complications that develop.

Thumb sucking is more than Just a Simple Habit. It is a multi-faceted complex pattern that can affect mind and body. Chronic thumb sucking can cause more than misalignment of the teeth. Every body part is connected, when chronic thumb sucking persists dysfunctions may develop due to other body parts adapting and compensating when normal functions are disrupted.

Parents, Patients (thumb suckers) and Professionals all have key roles in thumb sucking elimination. When parents have thumb sucking concerns. **Two Thumbs Up** provides a guide to discuss, interpret, process possibilities, expanding insight and decision making.

Professionals; the health care specialist and allied health care professionals are sought out by parents looking for answers, guidance and help. **The Professional Connection** chapter provides detailed information regarding the structural, functional and chemical changes that occur from chronic sucking patterns and how these changes affect your patients when not addressed. Two established thumb sucking elimination techniques are presented describing and comparing, a habit breaking appliance and behavior modification, their pros and cons. A sample step by step program is also presented including therapeutic protocols, strategies, helpful hints and pitfalls to avoid that may help therapists beginning their allied health care career. When parents/patients/professionals connect information, recognition and treatment the result is what she likes to call, **Total Patient Care.**
Desire + Awareness + Education = SUCCESS!

Chapter 10

Resources

Stories play a vital role in the growth and development of children. They build confidence, language and learning. Reading stories, a child can relate to, is a good first step to initiating a dialogue on the subject. Many children that are chronic thumb suckers develop multiple emotions; embarrassment, frustration, fear that they can't stop. 'Subject' education helps the child to obtain, to process, and to understand basic information needed to make decisions.

Storybooks that talk about thumb sucking may provide a pleasant fun approach to awareness of thumb sucking and education about thumb sucking elimination.
https://www.writersbureau.com/writing/Why-are-stories-important-for-children.htm

Storybooks provide 'Subject' Education in a Non-Threating Fun and Entertaining Way

Heitler, Susan M. Ph.D. **"David Decides About Thumb Sucking."** 1996. *May. Reading Matters, Denver CO.*
David sucks his thumb is a question/answer book. He tells how he feels, what questions he asks, tells what problems can occur when thumb sucking, conversations with siblings about the thumb, talks about what could be done to stop sucking the thumb, as well as, making the decision to stop sucking the thumb. There is a section for parents that answers questions regarding thumb sucking, concerns, help, and references. The book also includes programs of recording progress and rewards.

Berenstain, Jan. & Berenstain, Stan. 1987, August 12. "The Berenstain Bears & the Bad Habit." *Amazon*
We all love the Berenstain Bears, therefore, most children will love reading and relate to having a similar habit as their beloved Berenstein Bears. A good addition when a discussion about a bad habit needs to take place.

Wilkinson, Charles.1978. March **"The Dumb Thumb."** *Academy Press Limited.*, Chicago Ill.
A simple book that talks about feelings through the eyes of a thumb (figuratively speaking). This story is about a little boy, making it very easy for a male thumb sucker to relate to.

Ernst, Kathryn F. 1975. Oct. **"Danny and His Thumb."** *Prentice-Hall, Inc.* Englewood Cliffs, N.J.
Simple, kid friendly book, boys will relate to. Talks about all the different locations Danny sucks his thumb and what activities he can do when not sucking.

Dragan G. Antolos Dr. 2004. **"The Little Bear Who Sucked His Thumb."** *Dragan G Antolos*. Third Edition.
This story illustrates the emotional roller coaster a child experiences when sucking his or her thumb. It shows you can successfully eliminate thumb sucking with determination. The story emphasizes it is the thumb sucker's responsibility to want to stop thumb sucking to have successful thumb elimination. A positive approach is presented throughout the story. www.oliverthebear.com

Reference Books:

Gelb, H. D.M.D (1977) "Clinical Management of Head, Neck, TMJ Pain and Dysfunction," *W.B. Saunders Company.* Philadelphia/London/Toronto.

Hanson, M.L. PhD & Barrett, R.H. B.A., *(1988)* "Fundamentals of Orofacial Myology." Charles C. Thomas. Springfield, Ill.

Enlow, D.H. PhD (1975). "Handbook of Facial Growth." *W.B. Saunders Co.* Philadelphia/London/Toronto.

Hanson, M.L. PhD., & Barrett, R. H. B.A., (1978) "Oral MyoFunctional Disorders." *C.V. Mosby Co.* Saint Louis.

Hanson, M.L. PhD. & Mason, R.M. DMD PhD. (2003) "Orofacial Myology International Perspectives." *Charles C. Thomas LTD*, Springfield, Illinois.

Appleton, N. PhD. (1988) "Lick The Sugar Habit Sugar Addiction Upsets Your Whole Body Chemistry." *Penguin,* Barnes & Noble.

Fisher, J.E. & O' Donohue, W. T. (2006) "Practioner's Guide to Evidence-Based Psychotherapy." *Springer,* Reno, NV.

Milkman, H., & Sunderwirth, S. (1987) "Craving for Ecstasy: The Consciousness and Chemistry of Escape." *Sage Publications,* Thousand Oaks, California.

Proffit, W.R., Fields, H.W. Jr., & Sarver, D.M. (2006) "Contemporary Orthodontics." *Fourth Edition Elsevier Health Sciences.*

McKeown, P., (2004) "Close Your Mouth-Buteyko Breathing Clinic Self Help Manual." McKeown, P., Galway, Ireland.

Articles:

Phillips, C.J. Dr. (2014) "Positive Effects of Thumb Sucking after Birthing Process." *Excerpt from the Missing Piece* Source: ICA Cranias
    http://hol-solutions.blogspot.com/2014 could-thumb-sucking-past-age-of-3-be.html.

Sears, W. M.D. (2008) March 6. "Ask Dr. Sears: Thumb Sucking." *Parenting Magazine.*

Cettina, T. (2008) March 6. "Dealing with an Older Thumb-Sucker, Ways to help her kick the habit." *Parenting Magazine.*

"Digit Sucking - An Area of Benign Neglect." (1984) *I.J.O.M.* 10:33-36.

Van Norman, R.A. "Digit Sucking Children". *DVD - from lecture given at C.O.M. Midwinter conference in Law Vegas.* Forty-seven-minute lecture about the problem of digit sucking. Information, research studies, before and after photos, and highlighting ground- breaking work by orofacial myologists in this area.)

Van Norman, R.A. C.O.M., "Digit Sucking: It's Time for an Attitude Adjustment or A Rationale for the Early Elimination of Digit-Sucking Habits Through Positive Behavior Modification". *International Journal of Oro-Facial Myology, Volume 11 Number 2.*

Salah, A. Dr. BDS, MSc. "Mothers' Attitude Toward Digit Sucking Habits in Children of United Arab Emirates". *International Journal of Orofacial Myology.* 2007: Vol. 33. Pages. 37-45.

Research Articles: Research-Durham University

Reissland, N., Francis, B., Aydin, E., Mason, J. & Schaal, B. (2013)"The development of anticipation in the fetus a longitudinal account of human fetal mouth movements in reaction to and anticipation of touch." *Developmental psychobiology.* DOI: 10.1002/dev.21172.

"Babies learn to anticipate touch in the womb." *ScienceDaily.* 2013: 8 October.
    www.sciencedaily.com/releases/2013/10/131008091727.htm

"Practice makes perfect for thumb sucking in the womb." *The Times* https://www.thetimes.co.uk/article/practice-makes-perfect-for-thumb-sucking-in-the-womb-lx7n28qz3hq

Popovich & Thompson. (1973) "Thumb & Finger Sucking Its Relation to Malocclusion". *AM.J. Ortho.*, pp.   63-148.   Dent. Practice, 9:57, 19580- by Leech.

Bibliography

Nowak A.J., & Warren, J.J. (2000) "Infant oral health and oral habits." *Pediatric Clinics of North America*, 47 (5) pp.1043-1066.

Van Norman R.A. (2001) "Why we can't afford to ignore digit sucking." *Contemporary Pediatrics.* 18:6 pp.1-81.

"Quitting thumb sucking and pacifiers." *American Academy of Pediatrics:* 6/20/06.

Salah, A. BDS, MSc. (2007) "Mothers' Attitude Toward Digit Sucking Habits in Children of United Arab Emirates*." International Journal of Orofacial Myology.* Vol.33.

"Treatment of Thumb Sucking: An Analysis of Generalization and Side-Effects". (1987) *Journal of Child Psychology and Psychiatry and Allied Disciplines.* 28(2) pp. 281-95.

Graber, L.W. (1981) "Psychological Considerations of Orthodontic Treatment." *In Psychological Aspects of Facial Form, Center for Human Growth and Development.* University of Michigan, Ann Arbor, Michigan. pp. 81-119.

Made in the
USA
Middletown, DE